JUNK & FOODS
JUNK & MOODS

STOP CRAVING AND START LIVING!

Gloria —
You are awesome!
Hope this book
helps you on your
journey!

♡ Lindsey

This book was written and published in
partnership with inCredible Messages LP
www.inCredibleMessages.com

JUNK & FOODS JUNK & MOODS

STOP CRAVING AND START LIVING!

Lindsey Smith

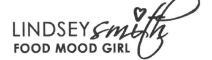

To contact the publisher, visit
www.inCredibleMessages.com

To contact the author, visit
www.FoodMoodGirl.com

Printed in the United States of America

ISBN-13: 978-0984798339
ISBN-10: 0984798331
Self-Help / Motivational & Inspirational

Cover photo: Scheller Image and Design

Cover design: Amie Olson

Book design: Amie Olson

Styling: Aire Plichta

Special thanks to Sugar Café in Dormont, PA for letting us film during business hours. Your kindness and gratitude are much appreciated!

Everything you want—you already have,
and everything you want to be—you already are.

*To all those who have been looking to food
for all the wrong reasons; my hope is that this book
feeds you with the exact nutrients you need!*

Contents

Acknowledgements

My Mentor, Ted Cibik

Thank you for instilling powerful basic principles within me at such a young age. With your help and support, I truly started to love and appreciate myself and gain vitality and health. Thank you for continuing to do the work that you do and believing in another way of living. Your passion shines through and it is much needed in this world. I am forever grateful.

My Book Coach, Bonnie Budzowski

The magic of this book sparked because of you. You have been a true gem and you have helped make this book come to life. You have been more than a mentor, coach, and editor; you have been an inspiration and a friend. The passion for what you do is so apparent. We have connected in such a way that I know you truly understand where I am, and you have always been able to give me the exact nutrient I need!

Amie Olson

Thank you for always listening to me and being there to support me through the process of what is going on in my head to what I actually want to make happen. You have a true gift of helping others, in more ways than one! I want you to know how beneficial your friendship, both personally and professionally, has been to me! The spunk of the book came to life because of you and your gifts! I am so grateful to have you by my side!

Karen Soroka

Life coach, finance coach, but most importantly, a true friend. I know you are always there for me at the drop of a dime. Your friendship has been so important because it has been one of the first relationships in my life where I have felt a sense of support from someone so naturally. You know what it takes to be a true friend, and I appreciate all the phone calls, talks, and informal meet-ups! I know you always have my best interest in mind, and you are one of my biggest cheerleaders! Thank you!

Zach Adamerovich

Thank you for sticking by my side and supporting me throughout the years. Your friendship is unlike anything I have ever experienced. We have definitely grown together and challenged each other along the way. I can always count on you to keep me grounded and sane.

My Clients

You all rock. You inspire me in so many ways. I feel every person I have worked with is a complete reflection of who I am or have been at some stage in my life. We work together and strive together. Through your healing, you all also help me heal. Your stories, personalities, and passions keep me going every day. We have walked in such similar shoes, and I love knowing that we are on the journey together. Keep up the great work, and I hope this book will help you along your life-long journey to health and happiness.

Mom, Dad, & Kristin

You all have seen my highs and lows throughout the years. You have seen me change numerous times. You have witnessed my emotions, my struggles, and my low points. Despite it all, you still have an unconditional love for me. You have all helped teach me and shape me in some way for the better. I hope this book speaks to you each in a way that helps you understand not only me, but your own self a little more.

Love you all unconditionally!

Lindsey

1

The Airport Stranger

How a Stranger Transformed My Perspective on Foods & Moods

I arrived at the airport around two hours before my plane was to depart for a trip to New York City for a nutrition conference. At 7:30 a.m., you might have thought I was ready to run a marathon; I was energized and ready to go. I decided to get started on writing some new articles. I grabbed a cup of hot tea and sat down at a table away from the morning rush and dove into my writing.

I had tried to pick a remote location in the airport so I could concentrate and let my creativity flow. I chose a back corner where no one was sitting. There were windows so I could see the runways. Since this was June in Pittsburgh, the sun was shining brightly, and so was I.

Just as I began to settle into my task, I heard a woman yelling and screaming. Startled by the commotion, I jumped up to see what the fuss was about. Then a woman came stomping out of a nearby *"Employees Only"* door, screaming into her cell phone. I saw the face of a woman in her late forties, and the face was filled with stress, anger, and misery. I heard the woman complaining loudly about her boss, how much she hated work, and how ready she was to go home. Her face was red and crunched up, sad, and she filled the room with a toxic fog of negative energy.

The negative fog felt heavy to me, and I hoped the woman would leave the area and leave me alone. Her tirade was almost too much to handle.

Fortunately, the woman did leave, and she took her negative fog with her. I started typing again. A paragraph or two flowed perfectly, and I forgot all about the stranger I had just seen moments earlier.

Then suddenly I felt the room getting foggy once again. The negativity was so strong this time that I knew this woman had come back. I looked up to find her sitting across from me. This time, however, she was sitting with a tray full of calorie-infested processed foods.

Of all the empty tables in the room, the woman I wanted to avoid sat right in my line of sight at the next table over. There I was, looking directly at her. I tried to pretend that I was not staring at her or her tray of food, but I just couldn't help myself. Being a *"foodie"* and a nutrition coach, I was curious to see what she was eating.

My unidentified angry companion had the following items on her tray: a large Ben and Jerry's chocolate milkshake with whipped cream; a bowl of ice cream with whipped cream; and a Styrofoam container filled with a huge omelet and hash browns, drenched with ketchup. Mind you—this was at 7:30 in the morning.

Disgusted, appalled, and angry, I felt the urge to jump out of my seat, grab the stranger by the arms, and shake her, screaming, *"What are you doing, Lady? Do you not realize this food is killing you?!"* However, I decided to refrain from public embarrassment and possible arrest; instead, I shook my head and shrugged my shoulders.

As much as I wanted to turn away and return to my typing, I could not help but bluntly stare in awe at this woman. It was like driving past a wreck on the interstate; you want to slow down to see what's happening, even though you know you shouldn't stare.

I proceeded to watch my companion scarf down her food. She started with the small cup of ice cream and went on to consume most the items on her tray: slurp-by-slurp, bite-by-bite, and chew-by-chew. With each bite I cringed a little more.

Then, as I sat immersed in private horror at this woman's behavior, something disturbing happened. She took a break from eating the items on her tray and pulled out a lunch box cooler. I thought, *"Is this lady serious right now? More food? What else could she possibly be eating? She just ate enough calories for three days!"*

The cooler, in fact, did not contain food. Instead, it contained five prescription medication bottles. One by one, my companion lifted a bottle, took out some pills and swallowed them with her chocolate milkshake—all the while acting as if nothing serious was happening, as if she had not a care in the world. This behavior, it seemed, was like second nature to her. It was as if she were completely mitigating the poison she ate because she had some pills to take care of it.

I was enraged! Here was a person poisoning her body and then attempting to *"fix"* it by taking a handful of prescription medications. Did she even realize that her food choices were probably causing the diseases she was taking all the medications for? I was sure my companion had a blood pressure pill, a cholesterol pill, a stomach pill, and of course an anti-depressant to top it off. I was also sure that each disease was self-imposed by eating junk.

I realized, then, that my companion and I were the only two people in this section. I felt like this war between us was now *"on."* It was the nutrition coach versus the prescription chocolate milkshake lady at 7:30 a.m. at the Pittsburgh airport.

My eyes were glued on the woman at this point. I just had to see what she was going to do or eat next. With each moment, however, I was losing more of my composure.

I couldn't understand how anyone could treat her body with such disrespect. To binge eat when you know it's bad for you, when you are on multiple medications? This concept was totally foreign to me *(or so I thought)*.

Finally my companion finished her omelet and continued sipping the rest of her milkshake. It seemed like the tasteless reality show was over. I assumed the pain and torture of watching this poor woman kill herself with food and drugs was coming to an end. After all, she had finished everything on her tray.

Just then, the woman pushed her tray away and grabbed her lunch box cooler once again. I thought, *"Oh my, what else could she possibly be doing now? More food? More drugs?"*

Time seemed to slow, and I felt the commotion of the busy airport around me stop. Suddenly, everything in the room became blurry except for my companion. Slowly, as I watched, she opened the cooler and reached in. Her face seemed to cloud with fear, sorrow, pain, loss, discomfort, and overall unhappiness.

She then lifted up her shirt, rubbed her stomach with alcohol, and injected herself with an insulin shot. She was a diabetic on top of everything else. My companion turned her face to the side, as if she could not bear to look at the injection. As the needle penetrated, she took a quick jump and her face settled in defeat.

At 7:40 a.m. in the airport, I completely lost it. I began to cry uncontrollably in front of this complete stranger. This moment not only shifted my approach to my business, it shifted my heart. *My attention shifted from this woman's bad habits with food to the pain that must be leading her to seek comfort in calories.*

At this point, I was no longer angry, disgusted, or appalled by this woman. My judgment, criticism, and sense of superiority melted away. I now felt empathetic, remorseful, and saddened by what I had just witnessed.

I began to think about what may be going on in this stranger's life that was causing her to run to food as her comfort, as her friend to fill a void. She clearly was not happy with her job; she was overweight; and to top it off she was diagnosed with diabetes. What if at the end of the day, food was the only thing that made her feel good, that gave her a sense of hope and comfort? It seemed clear that food was filling the void of other factors in this woman's life.

As my judgment was replaced with compassion, I saw a reflection in this stranger of what I could have been. My childhood had come with a series of traumas that left me broken and bruised, the very things I could now clearly see beneath the surface of my airport companion.

As a pre-teen, I had suffered from general anxiety disorder. Shortness of breath, headaches, sweaty palms, weight issues, and stomach problems were symptoms of something much deeper happening in my life. I had low self-esteem, I was overweight, and I just felt lonely.

Lunch tables at my middle school signified groups or cliques. I sat at a lunch table with a bunch of popular girls. However, there were not enough seats for me at the table, so I ended up sitting by myself at the next table over. Although my seat was still next to the popular table, the distance felt like a gigantic gap to a sixth grader. These girls openly discussed their weekend plans and upcoming events, but I was never invited. I didn't really belong.

The popular girls might say to each other, *"Mary, are you coming to the movies with us this weekend? What about you, Jill?* And the names went on. Yet, they never invited me, Lindsey, who sat right beside them all year. I was left thinking there was something wrong with me.

As a pre-teen, isolation and rejection are hard issues to deal with. The insecurities, loneliness and low self-esteem I felt caused huge amounts of anxiety and stress in my life. While many teens choose drugs or alcohol, I chose food.

Food became my comfort, my drug. I could not wait until lunchtime to get my Twix Bar fix. I could not wait to hear the 3:30 p.m. school bell so my mom could rush me off to McDonald's or Wendy's so I could inhale my milkshake and value meal. When I was eating, I felt good. I felt joy. I felt like I had the friend I was missing, the looks I wanted, the body I dreamed of, and the peace of mind I'd die for. Food was my addiction.

Who was I to judge the airport stranger when I had experienced such a similar battle years ago? During my anxiety attacks, Twix Bar overdoses, and weight struggles, I too used food to fill the voids of negative self-image, minimal friends, and my overweight self.

I'm grateful to my airport stranger because the connection between ugly food habits and brokenness became clear to me in a fresh way when I watched her. The difference between her and me, however, was that the pain of my past no longer defined me and pulled me into destructive eating habits. *With the help of others, I was able to choose a new beginning, a healthier life. You can too.*

Since that day in the airport, I've seen the connection between food habits and brokenness (food and mood) validated again and again. My clients who struggle with weight invariably describe deep wounds that drive them to their destructive behaviors.

Now I know that weight gain is quite often the symptom of an underlying issue. Until you get to the root of the problem, the weight will continue to be an issue. You need to explore and understand yourself as a whole person to truly overcome food addiction. Once you understand the root issues, you need to understand that you do not need to be defined or controlled by past or present feelings, emotions, or negative thoughts.

Where I used to simply counsel my clients about food, now I walk with them as they explore the issues that sit deeper than food and drive them to certain behaviors they want to change. The essential message of *Junk Foods & Junk Moods* is that overcoming a food addiction is much more than counting calories and controlling portions. Our habits surrounding eating and weight control really stem from the mind, body, and spirit. Once we can realize why we are eating a certain way or struggling with a food addiction, we can truly be freed of our weight troubles.

Junk Foods & *Junk Moods* is an inspirational guide to the little steps we can take every day to overcome our painful wounds and to fill the void with love, friendship, relationships, and wholesome foods in order to live happy and healthy lives!

If you have overcome a food addiction, are in the process of overcoming a food addiction, or just want to learn some good tips, then this is the book for you.

Bon appétit! Feel free to over-indulge!

2

My Personal Journey

From Swedish Fishes to Healthy Dishes

My negative relationship with food started when I was four years old. I was outside with my peers at pre-school where we were all waiting for our parents to pick us up. This was back in the day when our parents drive up and display a bright yellow or neon green laminated sign with our names on them. The teacher or teacher's assistant would then take us to our parent and we would be on our way.

One by one each of my peers had a parent displaying a sign. Eric, Ben, Renee, Heather and the others were all picked up. A young child's eternity went by, and still no sign for me. Feelings of anxiety started to rise. Where are my parents? Are they okay? Did they forget about me?

By the time my parents showed up, I felt forgotten, neglected, hurt, and lost. It wasn't the first time this had happened. As I waited, the following thoughts raced through my mind: Why am I always the last one left? Don't they love me? Don't they care about me?

Finally, my mom came to pick me up. The moment I saw her, I started sobbing. Tears poured out and I began to scream. I couldn't seem to calm down.

In a desperate attempt to get me to quit crying and screaming, my mom did the only thing she thought would work. She took me to Don Manns, a local convenience store filled with penny candy.

Mom told me to pick out any candy I wanted. The bright colors and the rows of jars were enough to excite me, and my tears began to dry. I filled my brown paper bag with all the essentials— watermelon gummies, sour patch gummies, red Swedish fish, and flying saucers.

This play of emotions and consoling food became a routine. Every time my parents were late, I would be rushed off to get a quick sugar fix to make it all better. *My parents were treating my junk mood with junk food.*

This routine set me up for an unhealthy relationship with food at a young age. I began to associate feelings of hurt, neglect, and sadness with sweet foods for comfort. It seemed these foods could take away any negative feelings I was having. This candy, however, was never able to address the real problem—my need to be loved and remembered.

The damage occurred early, but it didn't show for years. My parents were good to my sister and me, and they made sure we were cared for. Except for the deep need to be remembered and loved, I had pretty high self-esteem. I was also thin and fit; I had neighborhood friends to play with; and I was pretty carefree with most things. I was a *"free spirit"* child who enjoyed and appreci-ated life.

Then fourth grade hit. Suddenly, I was no longer the little stick figure I used to be. I had gained some weight and basically quit growing in length. My face was chubby, clothes didn't fit right, and I became extremely self-conscious. I was up to 140 pounds, and I was less than five feet tall.

Back-to-school shopping went from being fun to being a traumatic experience. I remember a specific day my mom took me shopping for clothes during the summer before fourth grade. I walked into the store delighted at all the sparkly jeans, fun tops, and accessories.

As it turned out, neither the clothes the mannequins wore nor those on the racks looked good on me. My enthusiasm was quickly deflated. Rather than feeling excited about shopping and getting new outfits, I felt depressed, angry, fat, and ugly. Why couldn't I look like those other girls? I remember feeling different, like an outcast. How come everyone else could fit into these clothes and look nice, but I looked *"fat."*

Finally, I settled for the only thing that fit me in the entire store— sweatshirts and sweatpants. My entire wardrobe in grades four through six consisted of two sweat outfits: one was lime green and one was grey and pink. Sweats were the only outfits I felt comfortable in. They *"hid"* everything I was afraid of—my changing body, my low self-esteem, and my anxiety. I used the sweatpants as a way to mask my internal and external insecurities.

In the midst of all these body changes, my parents' carpet retail business became first priority in their lives, and my life got put on the backburner. They often worked long and odd hours, running the entire store between the two of them. It became difficult for one or both of them to leave the store. My feelings of neglect became deeper and more pronounced.

At just this time, I had my first speaking line in a play that my class was putting on. I was so excited—thrilled! Even though I was shy, I felt pretty cool about getting on stage and trying this acting thing out! I could not wait for my parents to see my big debut.

Unfortunately, the big debut was on a Thursday evening at 7:00 p.m., during my parents' late night at their store. My grandma drove me to school since my parents were working, but Mom and Dad kissed me goodbye and promised to be in the audience.

At 7:01 p.m., the curtains opened to an auditorium filled with people—parents, grandparents, brothers, sisters, friends, aunts, and uncles. My eyes went to the fourth row, about four seats over. I can still see this moment clearly in my mind. I remember what I was wearing, the lighting, where my grandma sat, what she was wearing—and the two empty seats beside her.

Ten years old, my first speaking debut, and I was completely let down. The thoughts mumbling through my head, *"Do they care about their business more than me? Am I not good enough? What am I doing wrong? Don't my parents love me enough to come see me? Am I not important enough? Why me? Why do they always do this to me?"*

In my distress, I might have begun to act out in violent, aggressive, or wild behavior, resorting to violence or drugs. Instead, I internalized everything, choosing food as my comfort, and becoming a complete perfectionist.

I realize now that the perfectionism stemmed from *"not feeling good enough"* for my parents. My unexamined hypothesis went something like this, *"Maybe if I get all A's, they will say something to me. Maybe if I join this activity, they will support me."* I was always hoping that if I did something well enough, great enough, and amazing enough, my parents would whole-heartedly want to be there supporting me, no questions asked and no worries about their business. I just wanted them to be there for me, present in the moment, and proud of my accomplishments, no matter how big or small.

With perfectionism, came extreme internal anxiety. I became anxious about everything, from my grades, to the activities I was involved in, to just being around people—everything was a factor in my anxiety. At the same time, I was also battling depression and low self-esteem. I didn't fully love myself and had a huge negative self-image that only added to the stress and anxiety. I lived constantly in a *"fight or flight"* mode.

This struggle with anxiety went on for quite some time. Just as I had turned to junky penny candy for comfort a few years earlier, I started relying on food more and more to lift my mood. Since my parents were *"always busy,"* they usually resorted to fast food because it was easiest for them. Eventually, I became addicted and couldn't wait to get my next *"Number 5"* at the drive-thru. I skipped the kid's meals and went straight for Extra Value Meals. Needless to say, I put on more weight, felt drowsy, and even more depressed.

I hid my internal struggle extremely well, and even those closest to me didn't know how badly I was hurting. I did not talk about my feelings much, as most kids don't, so I let all these emotions and feelings boil and internalize.

I remember asking my mom to be home-schooled at one point because I could not take all the stresses of school and day-to-day living. Still, I did not express the extent of how I was actually feeling. Each day added another couple drops to my bucket of anxiety and despair.

About a year later, in fifth grade, the breaking point hit and the bucket started overflowing. The internalizations finally externalized. I wound up in the hospital, dehydrated to the point where I couldn't keep anything down.

At first I thought I was just *"sick."* As I got older I realized that this *"sickness"* was really a result of many, many panic attacks I had over that past year or so. I hid these very well from my parents, teachers, and other caregivers.

Eventually, the panic attacks went from once a week to once a day. I remember begging to go to a therapist or a counselor. I needed help. I was overweight, depressed, struggling with anxiety, without friends, and feeling lost overall. *I didn't really know who I was.*

I finally convinced my mom to make me an appointment to see some sort of specialist. I still remember this lady's office and the set-up. Everything was perfectly placed and polished. Her desk was neat and organized. She was petite and very well put together. As I was sharing my emotions with her, I remember feeling extremely uncomfortable. I was unable to express the roots of my unhappiness. I went for a few sessions and after a short time, the specialist said I was dealing with high anxiety.

In my mind, I was just diagnosed with anxiety. There was a problem with me. I now had a label to fit how I felt.

So what did I do after this? I completely turned everything into my *"disease." I started letting my diagnosis define who I was.* Since it was now known, I acted out externally. If my mom would ask me to do something, I would be *"too stressed"* because my anxiety was kicking in. I now had an excuse for all my problems.

The anxiety, fears, and insecurities seemed to get worse with every day. I remember strategically planning the time I got to school each morning so I wouldn't have to walk in front of a crowd of students. I convinced my mom to drive me to school every morning because if she didn't, I would have been the last one to get picked up at the bus stop, which meant everyone on the bus would see me.

I was ashamed of how I looked and who I was. I never felt *"good enough."* Comparing myself to others didn't help either. After multiple panic attacks, being hospitalized, and seriously contemplating my life, I knew there had to be *"something"* else out there for me.

Meanwhile, my sister Kristin had been going to a wellness center in our hometown, and I watched as a real change occurred in her. She not only lost weight and was walking every day, but she started to glow. She started to love life. She started to be happy in her own skin. Who doesn't want those things?

I asked my mom if I could try out the wellness center. After all, I had tried many other things that hadn't worked. I remember feeling scared and timid as we pulled up to a building surrounded by beautiful trees, plants, and wildlife. It was peaceful and calming.

As I walked in the door, I noticed things I didn't understand at the time—a Buddha head, a Zen garden, and some other weird-looking statues. I gazed at everything, wondering what I had just gotten myself into. Then Ted walked in, with a magnetizing sense of calmness about him. I immediately knew this is where I needed to be. I wasn't sure if it was going to work, was still nervous, but deep down, I felt like I was already starting to heal.

I will never forget the first session I had with Ted. I spilled my heart to him, he talked a bit, and then he gave me a simple hand-out about *"eating colors."* He instructed me to choose colors when I was making meals and choosing foods.

Eat colors? Hmm, who knew it could be that simple, right? I took the handout home and started to recognize what colors I was (or was not) eating. I realized I was eating a diet of mainly bland colors, foods such as bread, pasta, meat, potatoes, and cheese.

I began to start recognizing and adding color to my meals. I tried to make every plate exemplify the colors of the rainbow. I added foods like purple grapes, orange carrots, and yellow squash to my diet. I became extremely good at creating new meals and trying new things once I accepted the value of different colored foods.

"Eat colors" was the first of the three main guiding principles Ted taught me that have helped me through my journey. *This first principle had to do with the body: Feed your body with colors and good, real food.*

Ted also taught me about the power of my own mind. He guided me to understand that I couldn't let my thoughts of having anxiety manifest and make me anxious. The fact that I could control my own mind was a hard concept to grasp during my teen years. I now realize it's a hard concept to grasp at any age really.

Ted taught me that our thoughts often control our outer selves. By letting my thoughts constantly be of anxiety, I was making my situation worse. I had to train my mind, which took practice, patience, and change. Ted helped me to believe this was possible and that it is an on-going journey as well. *This is the second principle that guides my life since working with Ted years ago: Feed your mind with uplifting and positive thoughts.*

Ted also encouraged me to find a spiritual outlet. Ted never preached a certain religion or spiritual outlet. He simply encouraged me to find my own outlet, whatever that may be. *The third principle goes deeper than calories and thoughts: Make it a practice to feed your spirit and above all, learn to love yourself.* Since I was growing up in a family that did not go to church and did not talk much about God or any other religious figure, following this principle was a bit difficult. But nonetheless, I set out on my journey of spirituality. Setbacks and all, I dove deeply into discovering what best suited me.

As we worked together, Ted constantly reminded me of these key principles. Of course, I had questions about which foods were healthy and which weren't. Ted answered my questions, but he maintained that living a healthy lifestyle, through mind, body, and spirit, isn't about a specific diet. As I worked with Ted over time, this became a natural part of me.

Upon embracing Ted's basic principles, my life completely changed. I went from the girl who could not walk onto a crowded bus or into a crowded room, to speaking in front of my entire high school. I went from an overweight, low self-image girl to someone with a healthier, positive outlook on who she was.

These changes, of course, did not happen overnight. I was not suddenly fixed by a fad or crash diet and my life was suddenly amazing. Within a short amount of time, however, I DID lose weight, increase my energy, and learn breathing techniques to help my anxiety. I was also able to maintain this new lifestyle because the three guiding principles touched my whole being—mind, body, and spirit. This new healthy way of living now became a part of who I was and now am. I learned how to *"feed and nourish"* myself in all areas of my life so I can live in balance and harmony.

I understand that I was extremely young to learn all these guiding principles. I'm not sure why they clicked easily for me. Some people go through their whole lives experiencing and reliving traumatic instances or replaying painful circumstances, never being able to truly feel liberated or freed of their fears.

My hope is that my personal journey and the advice you find in this book will help encourage and inspire you to take charge of your life and health by using the guiding principles of mind, body, and spirit to help overcome food addictions, release your mind of the word *"diet,"* and create a healthy way of living.

3

Breaking The Cycle

You Don't Have to Let Your Past Define Who You Are Today

When I began my career in the health and wellness field, I was excited to teach people about leafy green vegetables, grocery store shopping, and farmers markets. I wanted to teach people about making healthier food choices that would help change and transform their lives. After all, these things had played a huge role in my recovery, so I wanted to help others transform their lives through their food.

Gradually, I began to realize that teaching people about food is good, but it is not enough. Our problems with weight involve a complex picture of needing to fill the voids in our lives. My own personal story is an example of how food can be more than a source of nutrients. Food was my best friend. At the end of the day, food was there for me, soothing me when I hurt. It tasted good, providing all the flavors I loved.

Food didn't judge me; it didn't care how I looked or what I did. It never talked back. It never told me I was ugly. It didn't care how much I weighed. Food was just there, present with me and providing me with a self-assuring love that I wasn't getting from anything else. My story isn't much different from many I've heard. *"Food" is much more than stomach-deep for most of us.* I've encountered stories that resemble my own, embodied in the stranger in the airport, clients, and friends. I've come to realize that food comes in many different forms.

To be truly nourished and fulfilled, our bodies require many different nutrients. These include the essential vitamins, minerals, and amino acids most dieticians talk about. The physical forms of food we eat—such as apples, oranges, and pizza—provide one type of nutrient. Nutrients also come in non-physical forms of outside factors, including fulfilling relationships, meaningful careers, and deep spirituality. Everybody needs both types of nutrients. When we rely on food alone to nourish us, we become out of balance in many ways.

We get our lifelines and energy, not only from the physical forms of food, but also from the mental and spiritual forms of food as well.

When most people think about dieting or losing weight, they automatically think of cutting back on physical food. They attempt to cut calories, limit points, or give up sweets. After all, if you want to lose weight, you need to change the way you eat, right? Well, not necessarily. Having non-food factors in balance and harmony is just as important for achieving a healthy weight as is controlling what you physically eat and drink.

Think back to a time when you started a brand new relationship. Things were fresh, fun, and exciting. You could think of nothing but this person and how happy he or she made you feel. You felt like you were on cloud nine, and nothing could bring you down. This type of feeling gave you energy, and friends might have told you that you had a certain glow about you. You might have found yourself less hungry, or you may have even started craving foods like fruits and vegetables. Whether you realized it or not, the feelings around your new relationship were feeding you in a positive way.

In contrast, think of a time when a relationship ended badly. You felt discouraged, hopeless, and depressed. You wanted to curl up on the couch with a pint of ice cream and watch sappy movies on repeat. You might have found yourself binge eating or craving something sweet. In this case, your negative feelings around the relationship were creating cravings in you. You were craving nutrients, and you turned to sweet foods to get them.

In our society, we push sweet foods to fill all kinds of needs and provide all kinds of nourishment. For example, according the movies and television, how do all females mourn a break-up? With at least one pint of ice cream. And what do moms give the baby to stop crying? Lollipops. What do teachers give students for being good or doing well on tests? Treats, snacks, or pizza parties.

When we eat junk foods, we aren't usually eating for survival or to curb hunger; we tend to eat junk foods more for emotional reasons. We use food to provide rewards, cover up sadness, mask guilt, and enhance pleasure. My clients admit to eating as a result of stress, don't you? Many of my clients also privately tell me about deep-rooted issues that occurred in childhood that cause them to eat or crave certain foods.

We eat to solve problems that food can't possibly solve. To make matters worse, when we eat junk food that contains processed sugar, our bodies become addicted. The same thing can be said for foods high in salt or other additives. Once we have sugar or salt, our bodies want and crave more sugar or salt, leading to what can easily become a life-long addiction. In fact, junk food has such a foothold in most of us that we firmly believe junk food tastes good and healthy food tastes bad.

Junk foods don't make our bodies feel better, even in the short run. Shortly after eating junk, our bodies feel out of sorts. We gain weight from the junk, and then we start to feel even worse about ourselves. Often, even as we eat junk foods, we experience additional feelings of guilt or anxiety because we know we are deciding to eat foods that will ultimately sabotage us. Have you ever thought, *"Oh, I shouldn't have eaten that last cookie?"* or *"I wish I hadn't given in and ordered dessert?"*

The whole *"junk foods and junk moods"* pattern is a continuous

negative cycle, leading us to feel worse physically and emotion-
ally. But each of us DOES have the chance to make a change for
the better. Starting today, we no longer have to spin in the same
"junk foods and junk moods" cycle. Even if you've been addicted
to junk foods for years, you can change how your mind, body,
and spirit get the nutrients you need. You don't have to let your
past define who you are today! Take a step, a leap of faith, and a
journey into the real authentic you, who you were meant to be—
happy and healthy.

4

How to Get the Most from this Book

Begin Your Journey to a Healthier You

This book is set up to focus on the three main areas which *"feed"* us: mind, body, and spirit. The first section of the book will help you cleanse the clutter in your mind. The second section will help you consider foods you put in your body. The third section will help provide good nutrients for your spirit.

Each section of the book contains steps to implement in your life. Do not try walking in all the steps at once, or you will get overwhelmed. Instead, choose a step to implement during a week, two weeks, or even a month. See how you feel and what difference the change has made. As the initial changes you make become incorporated into your routine, try adding another small change from another step. Remember, you are embarking on a process and a journey to a lifetime of health, not a crash diet that will begin and end in a month.

This book is meant to help *"feed"* you and guide you so that you feel refreshed, more confident, and happier in your own skin. It is not a fix-it-all pill or a magic diet. This book is simply a guide to learning to live a happier and healthier lifestyle.

So stop right now. Take a deep breathe in and out. Begin your journey to a healthier you. Feel free to over-indulge!

5

Feeding Your Mind

Think Good Thoughts

"Thoughts become things...choose the good ones."
~ Mike Dooley

Your mind controls your every being. You don't have to tell your body to breathe or move or think. Your brain is on autopilot 24/7/365. The following steps are designed to guide you to feed your mind. You can choose your destiny and shine like you are meant to! Remember to start small, implementing one or two steps at a time. *Small steps equal BIG RESULTS!*

Step 1

Envision Your Life--Now Live It

Allow yourself to escape and indulge in a dreamland—where your life is perfect and exactly how you would like it to be. Create your ideal world, choosing whatever makes you happy: your dream car, house, soul mate, job, or anything else that brings you joy. Maybe your ideal life is having a maid to clean your house every day, or living right on the beach. Maybe it is simply having peace with your mom or dad again. No matter how big or small, envision each aspect of your ideal life.

Now take yourself back to reality—why can't your life fit your dreams? Envision your life and all the wonderful things it can bring, and then start living it. No one said you couldn't have exactly what you want, and you shouldn't feel badly about reaching for your dreams. Try living out your dreams—you might just be surprised at the outcomes. The key is to keep your vision and focus clearly in mind.

Trust me, with managing a business, a social life, workshops, speaking engagements, traveling, and writing a book, sometimes I get caught up in the little things and lose my vision. I found myself rather scattered for a while and I thought to myself, *"Lindsey, what is going on with you?"* Although I remained positive and continued morning mediations to calm myself down, it was apparent that something was just *"off."* I spent quite some time trying to figure out the problem.

Then, believe it or not, it all came together at a Chinese auction. Yes, that's right, a Chinese auction.

Let me explain.

My friend, Tara, had invited me to a networking function at a local country club. As I arrived, I noticed a beautiful set-up, and approximately 100 women chatting happily. I mingled, met a few wonderful women, and then made my way to the Chinese auction table. There were tons of beautiful prizes, and I was really excited to try to win something! I purchased a few tickets and put them in bags for gift cards, books, purses, trinkets, massages, body lotions, candles, and a basket of health goodies. There were so many great prizes; I could barely contain myself because I wanted to win everything!

As the night wound down, the event organizers were ready to finally pick the prizes. I felt like a little kid—so excited, hoping they would call my number. As they started, I was itching with excitement. I was sitting on the edge of my seat hoping my number would be called first. Then, the first few prizes came and went. When they got to a prize I really liked, I would shout, *"Oh I want to win this prize.*" Still—my number was not called. Then a life changing "*aha*" moment occurred. I begin to think about what prize I really wanted.

Earlier in the evening, I had dropped raffle tickets left and right, caught up in all the possibilities. Actually, there were some prizes I was okay with, some I liked, some I really liked, and some I loved! Now I asked myself, "*Okay, Lindsey, what do you REALLY want? What prize screams your name? What prize reflects you? Ultimately, what do you TRULY want?*"

As the numbers were being called out, I set my heart on a gift basket from a natural food store where I always shop. The basket had organic groceries, a re-useable bag, and a gift certificate. I had admired the basket early in the evening, and I REALLY wanted that prize more than any other.

I sunk in my chair, closed my eyes, and envisioned exactly what I wanted from start to finish. I thought of the woman calling my number. Then I "*saw*" myself receive the gift basket, bring it back to my table with excitement, take it to my car, up my apartment stairs, and finally into my kitchen where I put all the groceries away. As I pictured myself putting the groceries away, I felt excitement and joy for winning. I envisioned this all in my mind.

Finally, they were about to call the winner for the gift basket that I just envisioned winning. I said to the other women at the table, "*I know I am going to win this.*" They chuckled and said, "*Okay, Lindsey—you keep saying that!*" I smiled, and as the woman announced the winning number, everything seemed to slow as each number she called matched the number on my ticket. I won what I had completely envisioned.

When I got home, I realized I had solved the mystery of why I had been feeling "*off*" all week: My experience with raffle tickets was an exact reflection of what was going on in my life. Like many busy people, I had been putting my tickets into many different baskets of life. I needed to stop for a second and envision what I

REALLY wanted, trust the process, and allow the rest to fall into place perfectly. It became apparent to me that that I had to really clarify what I wanted out of life and not get bogged down by things that make me unhappy.

When you find yourself scattered and pulled in many different directions, ask yourself if you are caught up in all the small things in life at the expense of the big things you really want. Are you caught up in the clutter of life at the expense of the big picture? If so, take some time to envision your ideal life.

~~~~~~~~ Get Moving ~~~~~~~~

List your top three ideals that you would like to envision and focus on. Then list the details of each. Read these every morning and night and really focus in on them daily. What differences do you notice?

Example: My ideal job is a health coach. My ideal includes being my own boss, creating my own schedule, helping people achieve a healthier life, working with clients one-on-one, creating programs that will enhance the lives of others, etc.

My ideal _____ is _____.

My ideal includes: _____

_____

_____

_____

_____

_____

_____

_____

_____

My ideal _____ is _____.
My ideal includes: _____
_____
_____
_____
_____
_____
_____
_____
_____

My ideal _____ is _____.
My ideal includes: _____
_____
_____
_____
_____
_____
_____
_____
_____.

Step 2
Create a Vision or Dream Board

As children, we are taught to *"dream big"* and *"go for the gold."* At a young age, we compete in sports and strive to excel in school. We start out in life dreaming big, and sometimes we get let down. Then we dream big some more and get let down some more. Teachers, peers, and other members of society come in and tell us we aren't good enough, we aren't skinny enough, we aren't smart enough, and eventually we stop dreaming and stop envisioning our ultimate success. Our dreams become dark shadows in the night.

As children, many of us aren't taught how to stay positive and persevere in the face of disappointment. Instead, when things don't go exactly as planned, we stumble upon negative outcomes, circumstances and thoughts. We feel put down and we eventually fall to the ground, not possessing the coping skills on how to get up and excel. We let negative circumstances and experiences define who we become.

This is where a vision board comes into play. A vision board, which can be taught or started at any age, is an essential part to dreaming big. The sooner you begin the better.

Return to the dreamland you envisioned earlier. Transfer your dream to a board with pictures, quotes, or anything that reminds you of your ideal life. Maybe you want a new car, a new job, a stronger faith, or a new relationship. Post tangible objects, quotes, or pictures on your board to remind you of your ideal or desire. For example, if you want a new car, put the picture of a dream car on the board. If you want a new job, write out your ideal job description and put it on the board.

Move your dreams to reality by posting them in a prominent place. This will help you see and envision what you want on a daily basis! Seeing the dream in pictures helps the unconscious part of your mind to pursue the dream even when you are not thinking about it.

When I visited my parent's house shortly after I had started my business, I decided to take a look at some of my old papers, report cards, and projects. I found funny photos, old t-shirts, and book reports. Scuffling through the papers, I came across a 10 x 10 poster filled with pictures from magazines and quotes. I realized I had created a mini vision board in middle school.

I had forgotten all about the dream board project and was quite surprised my family still held on to the poster. As I looked at my "*dream career,*" I was shocked. I was currently living my eighth grade dream. A picture of two hands holding each other reflected the coaching I was doing; a person speaking represented the public speaking that was a part of my business; and a book pointed to the book you hold in your hands.

In eighth grade I had envisioned myself helping people, speaking publicly, and writing a book. I was currently doing all three. I could not believe it. Even at a young age, I was setting my path up for the future.

No matter how big or how small, dream it, envision it, and make it real. A vision board will help you see, every day, what you really want and what you are working towards.

Who said you can't dream big?

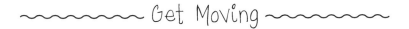

Get Moving

Create your vision board today!

1. Purchase a large poster board, dry erase board, or corkboard. Place it somewhere you can view it every day.

2. Fill the board with pictures from magazines, the internet, and newspapers. Use quotes, drawings, words, lists of goals, or anything that speaks to you. What are your goals? How do you envision your life? Include a picture of your dream car, a write-up of your ideal job description, and much more.

3. View your vision board every morning and every evening. Take time to notice each item on the board and envision yourself having it NOW!

4. Feel and express gratitude for what you already have.

5. Update as little or often as you like. Enjoy!

Step 3

De-Clutter Your Life to Reduce Your Stress

Do you have a mass of papers overflowing in your office? Is your closet a mess? Maybe you have a spare room where you store everything you can't find a place for? Believe it or not, this clutter could actually be adding additional stress to your life.

Our clutter reflects our reality. So if your office is a mess, chances are your workload is a mess, which can make you feel overwhelmed and stressed all the time. When I work with clients who say they feel displaced, anxious, or over-whelmed, one of the first questions I ask is, *"Do you have anything that clutters you?"* The answer is always, *"Yes."* Whatever form it takes, clutter adds stress to your life.

To decrease stress from clutter, start small by organizing a drawer or closet. Build small successes and then eventually tackle the bigger projects like your office or that spare room. You'll feel a sense of accomplishment as you make progress toward organiza-tion and a calmer lifestyle.

When you think about de-cluttering, look at all aspects of your life, not just the tangible objects you can organize or clean up. Do you have a relationship that stresses you on a daily basis? Are you hanging onto baggage from a past relationship? As hard as it may be, sometimes we must de-clutter certain relationships or instances from our lives. If we hold on to false hopes or dreams of people turning into the people we want them to be, we are often let down and clutter the emotional space needed for anything greater to enter our lives.

From personal experience, I know this all too well. I held on to an ex-boyfriend for six years, keeping him around when it was convenient for me. This choice did not allow for greater, higher quality relationships to enter my life. Once I cleared the path of this unhealthy relationship, a whole new world of possibilities opened for me.

When you de-clutter the tangible objects, unhealthy relation-ships, and even angry thoughts you turn over and over, you reduce the negativity and stress you carry around. You also make room for more positive events, circumstances, and people to enter your life.

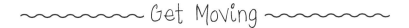

Get Moving

Start small with the tangible things, and build on your success. What are three areas of your life that you can start de-cluttering now? List them here and also list the action steps to make it possible!

Example: I am going to de-clutter my office. I will complete this by October 1, 2011. Here are the action steps I am going to take:

1. Start with drawer full of papers and go through all my papers and shred and recycle what I am no longer using.
2. Move to supply drawers and go through supplies. Throw out what I am not longer using.
3. Organize drawers to be systematic.
4. Go through books/CDs/DVDs and compile ones that I no longer use. Donate to Goodwill.
5. Put new books and old books organized on bookshelf.

I am going to de-clutter my _____. I will complete this by _____. Here are the action steps I am going to take:

1. _____

2. _____

3. _____

4. _____

5. _____

I am going to de-clutter my _____. I will complete this by _____. Here are the action steps I am going to take:

     1. _____

     2. _____

     3. _____

     4. _____

     5. _____

I am going to de-clutter my _____. I will complete this by _____. Here are the action steps I am going to take:

     1. _____

     2. _____

     3. _____

     4. _____

     5. _____

Step 4

When You Can't Change the Circumstance, Change Your Attitude

One evening, I got home weary from a day of back-to-back meetings. I still had to prepare for weekend events, submit a proposal to a client, and follow up on a ton of e-mails. I was facing a full evening of work.

I turned on my relatively new Macintosh to find that it was functioning slower than normal. Then, the computer completely froze. After a bit of troubleshooting, I rushed to the Apple store to see what was wrong. Sure enough—my hard drive had completely crashed. All of my business files, proposals, manuscript, pictures, writings, and marketing materials were on this computer. No back up at all! I panicked for about 30 seconds before saying to the technician with a smile, *"Okay, Dan, what can we do about this?"*

Despite experiencing what many of us would consider a major disaster, I remained positive. I thought to myself, *"Honestly Lindsey, what can you do about this? This is the card you are being dealt, and it makes no sense to get upset, freak out, worry, or flip out at the technicians."*

I had to think outside of the situation and ask myself, *"What is this situation telling you? Is it telling you to slow it down a bit? Is the lesson to make sure you always have a backup hard drive? What is the lesson here?"*

Even the most trying, inconvenient, and upsetting circumstances have a message for you. Sometimes you need to really dig deep to see the positive light in the situation. You might not know right away what hidden message or what positive circumstance might reveal itself, but there is always sunshine after rain. A new day always begins.

Life can be as amazing or as difficult as you want it to be. You have the power to transform the bad to the good. There is no sense getting upset or mad at situations that are out of your control. By getting angry or upset, you only attract more situations of negativity into your life.

Let's face it, I could not control or change my hard drive situation. I could not suddenly go back in time and bring back my hard drive. Nor could getting upset with Dan, the technician, make the situation any better. Instead, I chose to change my attitude, knowing that things would work out in the best way possible if I remained positive. And things did work out—and I learned a valuable lesson about backing up my files.

A way to overcome a negative response to situations is to stop yourself midstream, and take a deep breath. Once you calm down, begin to think positive thoughts. If it's hard to do at first, then try thinking back to a time when you overcame something really challenging. Tell yourself, *"Wow, if I got through THAT, how easy is THIS?"* Remind yourself and give yourself credit for obstacles and challenges you've already overcome.

Are you happy today? Only <u>YOU</u> have the power to control your attitude. So if you find yourself in a difficult or trying situation you can't change, try changing your attitude instead.

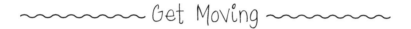

Get Moving

The next time you are feeling down or something bad happens, stop and tell yourself these positive affirmations:

I am complete and whole right now.

I love myself and I am an amazing person.

I have the infinite power to overcome anything that comes my way.

Insert your own here: _____
_____.

Insert your own here: _____
_____.

*"When the sun's not shining on the outside,
make it shine on the inside"*

Step 5

Allow Yourself to Grieve and Feel Your Emotions

We all experience times when we feel sad or upset. Unexpected situations break into our plans and our positivity. Sometimes it becomes hard to focus our minds positively because we are bogged down with tragedy. When this happens, remember it is okay to feel sad and to process your grief. You don't have to pretend everything is okay when it isn't.

In our society, we are often forced to wear a mask. Even in times of deep loss, we are only allowed a short amount of time to grieve. Then we are expected to return to our jobs and daily routines as if nothing has happened. This is true even when we lose a very close family member. Most times we are not given nearly enough time or space to process our emotions.

When we mask our feelings and emotions, they become bottled up, deeper and deeper. Eventually, we go down a path of self-destruction in some shape or form. Many people gain weight, become depressed, and become addicted to drugs or alcohol. Some even go as far as to hurt themselves.

The clients I have worked with regarding weight issues typically have a grief issue or underlying tragic event that troubles them. In nutrition coaching, I have heard stories about rape, suicide, death, bullying, anxiety, stress, neglect, torture, and abuse. These issues always point to the true problem. Weight problems or illness virtually always stem from a deeper issue.

I have worked with many clients who turned to food as their comfort during a loss or grieving time. Food became their friend, their drug, and their comfort through the rough times. Some who were victims of abuse used food to mask their bodies and appear more unattractive in the hope of avoiding attention. In each case, the weight and the food were merely the symptoms of the real problem.

Masking deep problems or our feelings about them only creates or feeds other symptoms. So if you are gaining weight or trying unsuccessfully to diet, focus on identifying and overcoming the root of the problem. Allowing yourself to grieve and get to the bottom of the emotional problem will help free your spirit and rid yourself of the negativity you have bottled up inside of you.

Once you recognize your root issue and can feel the emotions surrounding it, you can move forward productively.

Complete the following sentence, *"I am angry/sad/upset because. . . ."* Make a list and let all your negative emotions go! These negative emotions are only hindering your health! Release them and you will be free not only mentally and emotionally, but physically as well.

What is something that you haven't been able to let go? A broken relationship? A traumatic incident? A sad time?

~~~~~~ Get Moving ~~~~~~

In the space below, make a list of negative emotions that are hindering your health and happiness. Let the emotions you have kept bottled up come into the open. Let it all out! Allow yourself to feel your emotions that come as you complete the list. Then let the emotions go. Release them! You are one step forward to not only dietary success, but also emotional success!

I am angry/sad/frustrated/mad/upset/fearful/hurt/remorseful because _____

_____
_____
_____
_____
_____

———————————————————————————
———————————————————————————
———————————————————————————
———————————————————————————
———————————————————————————
———————————————————————————
———————————————————————————
———————————————————————————
———————————————————————————
———————————————————————————
———————————————————————————
———————————————————————————

Step 6

Increase Your Self-Love and Self-Acceptance

Insecurities—we all have them. While I am happy with myself and confident in my being, subtle doubts and insecurities creep into my mind from time to time.

I can think of many instances where I thought, *"I'm not doing enough."* *"Am I going to make it?"* *"I'm not skinny enough, pretty enough, nice enough."* And the list goes on.

Like you, I've seen countless billboards, TV commercials, and magazine advertisements to give me a kick in my own ego and want someone else's hair, body, or general looks. Our society constantly encourages us to search for something better than ourselves.

As a child and pre-teen, I binged on food to mask the pain of my deep wounds. Despite overcoming many obstacles and starting to live a life I enjoyed in my teen years, I still felt a sense of unworthiness. No matter how much I accomplished or excelled, I found an underlying sense of *"not good enough."* Even when I won an award or placed first in a competition, I still struggled with feeling inadequate.

This pain carried into college, where I binged on alcohol to mask the anxieties I felt before going out with friends. The alcohol, like food, was a form of self-medication. I eventually concluded that the overeating and the alcohol were not the root problem. The problem was my own lack of self-love. Despite the changes and progress I had made throughout the years, I had never embraced those changes or even appreciated and celebrated my successes. Instead, I felt a constant cloud over my head telling me I wasn't good enough. The source lay in my childhood, where deep wounds lay.

I'm certainly not alone in experiencing self-doubt when the facts say I'm unique, wonderful, and accomplished. Hands down, the underlying issue most people suffer from is denying their own self-worth. Internal doubts that creep into our minds and cause us to not fully love ourselves are widespread. Often, we seek nutrients outside of ourselves—a romantic relationship, a fancy purse, a bag of chips, or a drug. We crave these other nutrients to give us that feeling of love or security we are missing within. So how can we overcome this? What can we do NOW to wash away our insecurities and doubts?

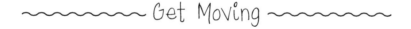

Get Moving

First things first. Remember, you are not alone! Everyone has these doubts, insecurities, and thoughts. Even the most secure people still get a hint of doubt every now and then.

Second—Start loving YOU! Many times we are so *"others"* focused that we neglect to take time to love ourselves. Do you treat yourself with the same consideration you offer to others? If not, start by making time for yourself, and doing things for you!

Lastly—start shifting your thoughts from the negative to the

positive. This sounds easy, but it can be challenging. So start small. When fears and insecurities creep in—keep telling yourself all the great things you have to offer.

With some practice, you'll not only say and do these things, but you'll believe them! If you find you are having trouble, or if you want to incorporate an affirmation into your daily routine, use this affirmation every morning during a quiet meditation time to help center yourself with self-love and self-worth.

In this moment:
> I am FREE.
> I am STRONG.
> I am ENOUGH.
> I am right where I need to be.

Step 7
Give Yourself an Attitude Adjustment

When it comes down to it—life can be hard. We lose loved ones, our workplaces are less than ideal, and we have imperfect relationships. Many of us lose faith in God, our families, and ourselves. We have trust issues, guilt issues, and intimacy issues due to past experiences in our lives. As the saying goes, everyone has a story. You can't choose all the circumstances that come your way, but you can choose how you respond to them.

One afternoon, I was at the grocery store during a chaotic time. When I got to the checkout line, I was surprised to find all ten lines that were open were backed into the aisles. I took my place in the self-checkout line and waited. People around me were sighing in disgust, checking their watches, and tapping their feet. Some people's faces were turning red and others frowned in anger. If looks could kill, a lot of people would have been dead!

I chose to smile, compliment the lady's purse behind me, and give off a carefree attitude. I was not going to let waiting in line a few minutes affect my day or my mood. I figured since I didn't want to join the angry crowd, I might as well try to lighten the air.

I became curious to see how long I would actually have to wait in line. Although it seemed like a long time, the actual wait was approximately four minutes. You heard me, only four minutes. People all around me were getting upset and angry over less than a ten-minute wait. Our society is so fast-paced and impatient that people blow out of proportion even minor inconveniences. This impatience is bad for our health and bad for our mood.

From our attitude about a wait in a checkout line, to our attitude about serious illness and death, we all influence how *"hard"* life is by the choices we make and situations we choose to get upset about. Practice making your life *"easier"* by recognizing those situations in which you get upset and asking yourself, *"Can I control this?" "Am I making my life harder with a negative attitude?"* Recognize the moment and appreciate the moment. Stop and just smile. Put yourself in a happier mood.

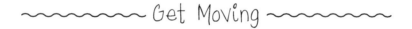

Get Moving

Practice your attitude! Check yourself in certain situations or scenarios by doing the following:

Assess your present attitude—does your attitude:

- Make you feel happy?
- Keep you on track?
- Make you feel good about life?
- Help you stay motivated?
- Help you smile?

If you answer *"Yes"* to any of these questions, then kudos to you! You have an awesome attitude! If you answer *"No"* to one or some of these, then stay calm and move on to the next step! (And remember, this is something we continuously must work on—our attitude may be good one day and *"junky"* another day. Always keep yourself in check!)

Start right now and indulge in a healthy attitude. Throw out the words *"can't," "not," "won't," "shouldn't,"* etc.

Change your negative words into positive ones—I CAN get through this, I WILL be happy, I AM amazing, I AM always on time, I CAN achieve great success, I WILL make it through this grocery line quickly!

Practice, practice, practice. As I mentioned before, this is something that we have to continuously work on—especially when situations are less than ideal. However, we have the power to practice and change our attitudes during trying circumstances.

Step 8
Get Uncomfortable and Grow a Little

I consider myself a shy person. I have an *"introverted"* personality, and I consider myself somewhat socially awkward. When I mention my shyness to others, the response is always the same—*"What, Lindsey? You, shy? I don't believe that. You are a motivational speaker and business owner, for goodness sake!"*

There is some irony here. I speak to audiences of all sizes and in all different parts of the country, sharing personal stories and personal struggles—yet, I'm shy? Yes, overcoming my shyness is something I work on every single day. It takes a lot out of me to network, put myself out there, and speak to audiences. However, I constantly push myself.

When I don't feel like starting a conversation with someone at a networking event, I do it anyway. When I feel shy about sharing a personal story, I push myself to do it. When in a huge line at the local coffee shop, I push myself to start a conversation with the person behind me, even if it means feeling uncomfortable in the process.

While growing up, withdrawing was comfortable and reaching out to others was extremely uncomfortable. Over the years, I started to realize how much I need to place myself in uncomfortable situations. Being uncomfortable means I have the opportunity to grow and push myself to places I never thought I would be able to reach before.

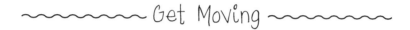

Get Moving

Don't let your mind deceive you into believing you should stay where things are comfortable for you. Starting today, practice being UNcomfortable! When you take yourself out of your comfort zone for a minute, for a day, for a week, it allows you to grow in an area you thought you could never grow in before. Try it! You might just be surprised at what you can do. Here are a few exercises to get you on your way:

List five areas in which you would like to see yourself grow.

1. _____

2. _____

3. _____

4. _____

5. _____

Now identify and write one thing that makes you feel uncomfortable about moving forward in each area. Identify a small uncomfortable step you can take to break the pattern. Try taking one step today, this week, or this month. Start small and work your way up. The more you step outside of your comfort zone, the more you will grow!

Feed Your Mind - Quick Mental Cleansing Tips:

- Envision the ideal life—then live it.

- Clean out a cluttered drawer or closet.

- You can't choose all the circumstances that come your way, but you can choose how you respond to them.

- Allow yourself to feel your emotions and grieve a situation, but don't let these emotions control your very being.

- Smile. Your smile will likely brighten someone's day, and yours as well.

6

Feeding Your Body

Eat Real Food

Let food be thy medicine and medicine be thy food.
                                        ~ Hippocrates

The food you eat is intricately interwoven with how you feel, whether you are aware of this or not. Here's how it works. The things you put into your body reflect what you are feeling on the inside. The things you put into your body also impact your feelings, creating a cycle. You get to choose whether to engage in a productive cycle or an unproductive one. For example, if you drink a large quantity of a caffeinated beverage, you are going to feel more jittery, stressed, and tense than if you drink a large quantity of water.

Your life CAN and WILL change when you put the right things in your body. This section covers steps you can take in your everyday life to enhance your nutrition and create a better sense of wellness.

Step 9
Incorporate Small Food Changes over Time

At a networking event for a women's group, participants around each table were instructed to give a 60-second commercial about who they were and what they did. Everyone had had a chance to express her commercial, and it was finally my turn.

Just as I was about to give my spiel, the MC announced that dessert would be coming around. Without thinking much about this, I continued to talk. In the middle of my commercial, the server came over and put the dessert tray right in front of me.

For some reason, no one at my table wanted dessert that night. Coincidence? I think not.

When it comes to eating, I am usually perceived as the *"odd ball."* People assume my diet is immaculate and become self-conscious about what they are eating or the food choices they are making when I am around. And while I consider myself healthy and very conscious of what I put it my body, I did not get like this overnight, nor do I judge others by their food choices. My encounter with the airport stranger cured me of that. I face facts: I'm not perfect. I enjoy a nice slice of cheese pizza now and then.

Healthy lifestyles are not created overnight. This does not mean you can't work at a healthy lifestyle and start incorporating small changes. Small changes over time will eventually pay off in big ways. Small changes make healthy living easier as each change gets incorporated into your lifestyle.

As Americans, we gravitate toward fad diets—because we want results yesterday! However, when we try to make too many lifestyle changes at once, we eventually crash and burn. Start small and the results will grow.

Keep Going

What can you change NOW? What are two to three things you could be doing for your physical health that you currently are not doing? Start incorporating one, two, or three changes in the coming week and notice the difference. How do you feel? Take notes.

This week, for my health, I am going to:

1. _____

2. _____

3. _____

Step 10
Treat Your Body Like a Test Lab

Do you feel energetic after eating an apple? Or maybe you feel full and satisfied? Or maybe you even feel bloated or tired? The food choices that work for your mom, your dad, or your friend might not work for you. Our bodies are unique; any given food has a different impact on each person. Foods that can heal you might hurt someone else.

When it comes to nutrition, treat your body like a test lab. When you eat something, notice how you feel after consuming that food. Does that specific food make you feel energized, lethargic, or gassy? Maybe the food energizes you at first, and then you crash later.

Answer these questions: How do you feel after a cup of coffee compared to a cup of green tea? How do you feel after eating an apple compared to a candy bar? It's important to experiment with your foods and your feelings. Dig deep into understanding your unique makeup!

It took me many trying experiences to genuinely pay attention to my body's reactions to food. I was so used to eating quickly that I failed to recognize how I felt afterwards. For example, early in life I got hooked on the habit of drinking coffee. It started with my first chocolate brownie Starbucks Frappuccino in eighth grade. Within a year, I was completely addicted to plain black coffee.

I knew coffee gave me a quick burst of energy—I felt perked

up, focused, and ready to conquer the world just after I drank one cup. I failed to notice, however, that I began to need more and more coffee to give me the same burst of energy. Caffeine is no different from any other drug; you grow to need more to give you the high you seek, and I was highly addicted.

Once I could no longer easily reach the high I craved, I began to feel extremely lethargic and drowsy. I also began to get frequent headaches. I even started experiencing acid reflux for the first time. Once I realized my coffee habit was making me feel lethargic and sick, I could make a decision about whether or not I wanted to continue the habit. The first step to kicking the habit was paying attention to my body.

Sometimes a food that leaves you feeling great in the beginning can lead to problems later on. You need to be aware and recognize these instances. It might take a little while for you to realize what is troubling you or why you feel a certain way after eating a certain food. Be your body's detective and try to de-construct your feelings. By doing so, you will be able to recognize and make healthier choices for the future.

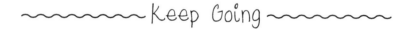

Keep Going

Try testing one of the foods on the following chart this week. Detect and record how you feel after eating each one. Keep track and notice patterns. This will help you gain a better understanding of what is or is not working for your body type specifically.

Type of Food	How did you feel right after?	2 hours later?
Dairy Milk, cheese, etc.		

Caffeine Coffee, sodas, tea, chocolate		
Meat Red, white		
Gluten Breads, crackers, pastas		
Citrus Orange, lemons, grapefruit		

Step 11

De-Construct Your Cravings

As humans, we naturally experience cravings. We crave everything we need in one form or another. For example, we crave foods, relationships, friendships, community, physical touch, and many other things. In itself, craving is not a bad a thing. When it comes to food, however, we have to know how to de-construct our cravings to know whether they are good for us or not.

The first step in de-constructing a craving is honing in even further with your detective skills for your body. You have to ask yourself the following questions:

- What do you crave?
- When do you crave it?
- How long have you craved it?
- When did the craving start?
- What is your mood before your craving?
- What is your mood after your craving?
- How satisfied are you when you give into your craving?
- How do you feel after you give into your craving?

Ask yourself these questions regularly. Often times, we crave something, but don't stop to see why. We either give in to our cravings and feel badly about it, or we don't give in and continue to struggle with the craving! Answering the questions above will help you understand what you are craving and why.

~~~~~~~~~~~ Keep Going ~~~~~~~~~~~

Once you assess your cravings, use the following chart to take your analysis a step further. Track your cravings for the next several days in the chart below. You can also visit **www.FoodMoodGirl.com** to download *The Two Week Food and Mood Chart*.

Date	Craving	When?	Mood Before	Mood After	Outside Factors? Stress level, relationships, etc.
1/1/12	Sweets	7:00pm	Bored	Tired	Stressed

After you complete tracking your craving patterns, use the following chart to de-construct your cravings even further. Use this chart simply as a guide. For example, if you crave sweet food, you might want to either cut back on your red meat intake, or you might want to work on improving a relationship in your life. Both of these *"feed"* you in a different way. A need in either area might be causing your sweet craving.

Common Cravings	What your body may really need:	Sample nutrients to incorporate:
Sweet Food	Natural energy Less red meat Detoxifying nutrients Less stress More rest Balance	Dark leafy greens Fruits Sweet vegetables Seafood Natural sweeteners More sleep/rest Quiet meditation Time with friends/family
Salty Food	Natural minerals Water	Unrefined sea salt Water, lots of it! Root vegetables Sea vegetables
Chocolate	Magnesium Balance	Raw nuts and seeds Legumes Fruits Natural sweeteners Exercise Stress reducing activities
Caffeine	Natural energy Less stress More rest Balance Detoxifying nutrients	Dark leafy greens Whole grains Raw nuts and seeds Legumes Raw fruits Exercise More sleep/rest
Bread/Pasta	Whole Grains Balance	Whole grains Raw nuts and seeds Legumes Time with friends/family

Refer back to this chart as often as you need to whenever you are craving a certain food or drink.

Step 12

Taste the Rainbow (No, Not Skittles!)

Colors are one of the most important factors to consider when choosing foods. Most people tend to eat plain and bland colors like yellow, tan, and brown. Foods with these colors are usually highly processed and contain the least amount of nutrients. Richly colored foods provide essential nutrients to keep you healthy. Each color serves a specific purpose in helping you function and stay healthy.

Red foods, such as apples, cherries, and radishes, help keep the throat and lungs strong.

Orange foods, like carrots, provide Vitamin A, which helps improve and maintain healthy vision.

Yellow foods, like bananas and squash, provide essential nutrients to help keep joints moving and pain free.

Green foods, especially dark green leafy vegetables such as kale, bok choy, and spinach, help stimulate new tissue growth and kick the immune system into high gear. Greens are also essential to weight loss, mental clarity, and enhanced mood.

Blue/Indigo/Violet foods, such as blueberries, grapes, and purple cabbage, help improve your heart and boost your memory. Feeling a brain fog coming on? Pop some blueberries and grapes into your diet!

~~~~~~~Keep Going ~~~~~~~

When you are making breakfast, lunch, or dinner this week, make a special effort to include more color into your diet. Who says you can't have spinach or kale for breakfast?

Check out the following recipes to see how you can include colorful food into your diet, every day and easily.

Super Original Green Smoothie

This smoothie can be used as an energizing breakfast
or a mid-day pick me up!

Side effects include increased energy, reduced cravings, and a positive attitude.

Ingredients:
- Handful of your choice chopped greens
  (Spinach, kale, dandelion, or another favorite green)
- 1 Banana
- ½ cup Almond or Rice Milk

Directions:
Blend well in blender. Add ice for a thicker texture. Serve immediately.

Note - You can also try adding other fruits and vegetables to add more colors! Make it fun and make it your own!

The first piece of advice my mentor shared with me as a kid was simply, "Eat colors." I thought I was there to talk about my anxiety and weight issues and he told me to just focus on eating colors. As simple as it sounds, it drastically changed my life! If you allow it, it can change yours too!

The "Other" Super Original Green Smoothie

This smoothie can be used as charging breakfast or after dinner treat!

Side effects include reduced cravings, satisfied appetite, and a positive attitude.

Ingredients:
- ½ an Avocado
- 1 Banana
- ½ cup Vanilla Almond or Rice Milk
- 1 tablespoon raw cacao
- 1 teaspoon fresh chopped mint

Directions:
Blend well in blender. Add ice for a thicker texture. Serve immediately.

Step 13

Check Your Sweet Tooth

Okay, so I admit, I used to be a sugar addict. It all started with those watermelon gummies. Quickly, I upgraded to Twix bars and eventually I found myself hooked on Chocolate Brownie Frappuccinos. It seemed like every year, I upgraded my addiction to the newest sugary treat.

After all, sugar consumes us on a daily basis. It is in almost everything we eat or drink. Sometimes it is seen as the basic word, "sugar" and sometimes it is disguised as high fructose corn syrup, dextrose, lactose, sorbitol, or sucrose—just to name a few! Despite the many names, the verdict is still the same—it's all sugar!

Sugar, in a refined form, can take our body on an emotional roller coaster ride. When we first digest it, we get this jolt or high. We may become extremely anxious or excited. Then, the ride dips and our anxious or excited emotions turn to depression or fatigue.

In order to get out of our slump, we often will again, turn to sugar to give us a quick fix. This is a continuous cycle of junk foods and junk moods.

Even just a small amount of sugar makes us desire more. Over-consumption of processed and refined sugars can lead to weight gain and other serious health conditions.

~~~~~~~~~~~ Keep Going ~~~~~~~~~~~

So instead of using table sugar or even artificial sweeteners, try slowly swapping out for natural sugar alternatives when you are cooking or baking. These alternatives are still sugar at the core, but they have a slower absorption rate in your body, so you most likely won't experience the emotional roller coaster ride that processed sugar takes you on.

Here are some natural sugar alternatives to try:

- Stevia
- Honey
- Date Sugar
- Agave Nectar
- Brown Rice Syrup
- Barley Malt
- Maple Syrup
- Molasses
- Unsweetened Applesauce
- Fresh fruit juices

*Note: These sweeteners are still to be used in moderation and merely as an alternative. The overall goal is to start to eliminate the constant need for sugary treats. These alternatives are a great way to help you wean yourself off the highly processed, refined sugars.

However, the overall goal is to start appreciating the sweetness of life, the sweetness of real fruits and vegetables, and the sweetness of being you. Eventually sugar alone will no longer be your main source of sweet.

Cripsy Nutter Squares

Ingredients:
- 1 cup brown rice syrup
- ½ cup almond or peanut butter
- ½ cup chocolate chips (recommend using the barley sweetened chocolate chips or carob chips)
- 3 ½ cups brown rice crispies cereal

Directions:
1. Heat brown rice syrup and almond or peanut butter in medium size pot, over low heat until creamy.
2. Stir in the chocolate chips until they melt in.
3. Remove from the heat
4. Pour the brown rice crispies into a separate bowl and pour the mixture on top.
5. Stir in until all brown crispies are covered with the mixture.
6. Gently press into a baking dish and allow mixture to set until firm, about 30 minutes.
7. Cut into squares and enjoy!

Chocolate Chickies

Ingredients
- Canola, sunflower or unrefined coconut oil
- 15 ounces (1 can) garbanzo beans, drained and rinsed
- 1/2 cup brown rice syrup
- 1/2 cup unsweetened apple sauce
- 1/4 cup almond or peanut butter

- 2 teaspoon. vanilla extract
- 1 teaspoon cinnamon
- 1/3 cup ground flax seeds
- 2 tablespoon brown rice flour
- 1/2 teaspoon baking powder
- 1 cup chocolate chips (recommend using the barley sweetened chocolate chips or carob chips)

Directions

1. Preheat oven to 350 degrees.
2. Lightly coat an 8-inch baking pan with oil.
3. Combine all ingredients, except chocolate chips, in a food processor.
4. Blend until smooth.
5. Pour the batter into the pan and stir in the chocolate chips.
6. Bake for 35-45 minutes, until cooked through.
7. Cool to room temperature on the counter
8. Enjoy!

Step 14

Keep Grocery Shopping Under Control

Grocery stores are now full-out marketing machines. You can't walk into a store for vegetables and bread without being bombarded with all kinds of unwanted stimuli: coupons, today's deals, fancy new products, a bank, a pharmacy, and/or a tempting café.

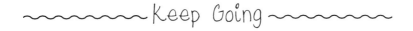

Keep Going

Here are some simple but effectives tips to help you make wise choices when grocery shopping:

- **Shop when you're full or satisfied, not when you're hungry.** When we are hungry, we make impulse purchases to satisfy our cravings in the moment. We end up spending more money and consuming more calories in the process.

- **Write a list and stick to it.** A list helps you to avoid running into the grocery store for three items and coming out with five bags.

- **Shop the perimeter or edges of the grocery store**—that's where about 97% of your food should come from. The processed foods (junked up foods) are shelved in the center aisles.

- **Do more of your shopping locally!** Take a trip to your local farmer's market or plant your own garden. This not only saves you money; it also cuts down on pesticides and contamination.

- **Skip the hurried shopping.** When we are running late, we often do our grocery shopping *"on the fly."* When you're in a hurry, you can't think about what you have in the house, what you want, and what recipes to make. Instead, you tend to choose frozen foods, chips, and other convenience foods. Discipline yourself to shop when you are relaxed and have your list ready to go!

- **Put your blinders on.** It's easy to get caught up in coupons, deals, free samples, and the latest *"weight loss"* endorsed products. Remember, these products have to move off the shelves without a salesman, so the manufacturers will do anything to increase a product's appeal to consumers. Put on your blinders and try to ignore the advertising.

Step 15

Understand Grocery Store Marketing Tricks

Since America has turned onto somewhat of a *"health"* kick recently, retailers and grocery stores alike are adding new *"healthy"* items geared towards consumers' wants and needs. However, when grocery shopping, it is easy to get confused about what is actually healthy. After all, most foods on the shelf originate in the mind of the marketer. Advertisers know the tricks to make you think you are buying a healthy option, when in reality, you may not be.

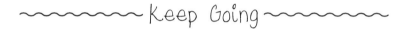

Keep Going

Here are the most common grocery store tricks:

- **Lightly Sweetened:** This simply means sugar is either being replaced by a substitute or the serving size is smaller. Sugar will be replaced with high fructose corn syrup or the serving size will drop to one cup rather than one and a half cups, thereby tricking the consumer into thinking the item contains less sugar when it does not.

- **Good source of:** This phrase is commonly seen on packages of cereals such as Cheerios, Golden Grahams, etc. "*A good source of*" simply implies that the food contains a serving of a certain grain. Advertisers fail to mention that you might have to eat an entire box of Cheerios to get the recommended serving of the *"whole grain."*

- **Multigrain:** More and more people are starting to understand the importance of eating whole grains. Many chips and snacks labeled *"multigrain,"* however, are highly processed. *"Multi-*

grain" simply means you'll find more than one grain on the ingredient list. You might think you are eating many grains, when you could be eating mostly white flour and bran. Be careful.

- **Reduced Fat:** In products such as crackers or microwavable meals, you will often find *"reduced fat"* on the label. However, the packages fail to tell you that the fat is actually substituted with sodium and sugar. Depending on your dietary needs, this information can be very important.

- **Natural:** A HUGE misconception surrounds this simple word. As more and more people are choosing organic, advertisers are putting the word *"natural"* into the mix. *"Natural"* has no standard in federal guidelines. In fact, many processed and refined foods can be considered natural because one ingredient came from Mother Earth. A great example is peanut butter. Since it is made from peanuts, it can be considered *"natural,"* even if it is loaded with sugar. Always look for the USDA organic labels to ensure quality.

- **Reduced Sodium:** The labeling practice around sodium is very similar to the one around *"reduced fat."* A lot of the time the sodium is reduced, but it is then replaced with fat and sugar.

- **Trans-fat Free:** A lot of marketers put this label on their foods. However, make sure you read the label carefully. Technically, products are considered *"trans-fat free"* if they have less than .25 grams of trans-fat per serving. The recommended maximum amount of trans-fat is 2 grams per day. So if you purchase a *"trans-fat free"* food that contains .25 grams of trans-fat per serving and eat the whole box, chances are you will have exceeded your amount of trans-fat for the day.

- **Only 90 calories:** Many packages say only *"90 calories"* or only *"100 calories."* However, the package size can lead you to believe you are eating less than you are. Many *"100 calorie"* packs are actually two serving sizes, which makes the entire package actually 200 calories, not 100. In addition, these products are typically versions of your favorite *"junk foods."* Unfortunately, the ingredients don't magically become healthier when the package size gets smaller. Fewer calories represent only one part of the healthy eating equation.

- **Whole Wheat:** Many companies put *"whole wheat"* on the labels of products such as breads, crackers, and chips. However, if you look at the ingredient list, the first ingredient is typically called *"enriched wheat flour."* This is just a fancy term for white flour. So even though you think you are eating *"whole wheat,"* you are actually eating white flour. Look for products that say, *"100% whole grain"* or ones in which the first ingredient is *"stone ground whole wheat"* to ensure you are eating the whole grain.

Our lives CAN and WILL change when we put the right things in our body. Try making one positive change for your body today. Home cook instead of eat out. Pick the fruit over chips. Start small and notice the changes!

Labeling Checklist

When it comes to food labeling, it is easy to get confused about what's healthy and what is not! Here is a simple way to read a food label without getting caught up in percentages, numbers, and all that other stuff. Of course, depending on your diet, you will want to pay attention to specifics such as sugar, salt, fat, protein, and calorie intake. For general purposes, three simple steps can rule a lot of unhealthy food out from the beginning!

1. What is number one? The first ingredient listed on the label is the ingredient of highest volume in any product. If the first ingredient is not what you want to eat, then don't buy the product! For example, if sugar is the first ingredient in a granola cereal, you are basically eating sugar, not granola.

2. If you can't pronounce the name of an ingredient, don't eat it! Simple enough.

3. If a product sounds too good or healthy to be true, it most likely is. After all, whole foods like fruits and vegetables don't need a convincing label on them for you to know they are healthy.

Stock Your Pantry with Healthy Staples

One of the most common questions I get is, *"What should I even buy?"* or *"What's even good for me?"* Even though the answer depends on you, your lifestyle, and your exact tastes, I have created a list of healthy staples that suit most palates to keep in your pantry. These staples, mixed with fresh ingredients, can be made into delicious meals, sweet treats, or easy dinners.

Use this checklist to ensure you have all the pantry necessities for healthy living:

Condiments

Oils: Extra virgin olive oil, coconut oil, canola oil

Vinegars: Red wine, balsamic vinegar, brown rice

Tahini

Tamari Sauce

Salsa

Honey

Agave Nectar

Seasonings

Sea salt

Fresh ground pepper

Dried herbs and spices

Pure vanilla extract

Canned Goods

Canned beans and lentils

Canned tomatoes and tomato paste

Broths

Grains & Legumes

Brown rice

Couscous

Whole-grain and rice pastas

Barley

Rolled oats

Dried lentils

Quinoa

Baking Products

Whole-wheat flower

Brown Rice flower

Quinoa flower

Almond flower

Baking powder

Baking soda

Nuts, Seeds, and Dried Fruit

Assorted raw nuts

Dried apricots, dates, cranberries

Nut butter

Step 16

Go Vegetarian for a Day

Many people laugh at this advice and respond, *"Oh, I could never give up meat."* In fact, there was a time I would say the same thing. I am not, however, asking you to give up anything! I am suggesting you simply try a new experience.

Try being a vegetarian for a day and see how you feel afterwards. Meats give our bodies a different feeling than fruits, vegetables, and whole grains do. Comparing a day without meat to a typical day with meat will provide valuable insight into how your own body functions. Experimenting as vegetarian occasionally will also help you to incorporate new foods into your diet, especially more fruits and vegetables.

Our palates are often pre-conditioned to eat what we ate as children. Those of us who grew up on fast food, convenience food, and junk food generally have a taste or craving for sweet and salty foods. Because of this, we've lost the craving for natural flavors that fruits, vegetables, and whole grains give us.

～～～～ Keep Going ～～～～

Try taking one day next week to go meatless. See how you feel. What differences do you notice? Take notes and try the experiment again! The more you become aware of how you feel after you eat specific foods, the better in tune you will be with your body, and the better choices you will make!

Don't know where to start? Here are five things you can do to experiment with going meatless for a day or two, or even a week:

1. **Start small!** There is no need to go out and purchase everything with a *"vegetarian"* or *"vegan"* label. Simply start back

to earth, with fruits, vegetables, grains, oats, nuts, and legumes.

2. **Adapt your favorite recipe the meatless way.** Use meat-free products such as tofu, tempeh, or seitan to adapt your favorite dish. You might also consider finding a recipe for a vegetarian version of your favorite meal.

3. **Try something new.** Next time you go grocery shopping, check out a meat alternative, a new grain, or a new vegetable. Consider this an adventure and enjoy seeing everything that is available.

4. **Buy a vegetarian cookbook or search for vegetarian recipes online.** Try one new recipe a week and discover what you like and what you don't like. Don't disregard a recipe if you don't like it the first time. Make tweaks where you feel necessary and try it again.

5. **Explore global foods!** Expand your palate and enjoy Thai, Chinese, European, and African food. Many cultures embrace a vegetarian lifestyle, so pull from these cultural traditions. You might find a new favorite dish!

My favorite EASY vegetarian dishes:

Vegetable Fried Rice

Ingredients:
- 1 small onion, chopped
- 1 tablespoon olive oil
- 2 cloves garlic, minced
- 1 carrot, diced
- 1 red pepper, chopped
- 4 cups cooked long grain brown rice
- 2 tablespoons tamari soy sauce
- 1 teaspoon toasted sesame oil
- 1 organic, cage-free egg (optional)

Directions:

1. Sauté onion in olive oil for 5 minutes.
2. Add garlic, carrot, red pepper, and sauté for 5 minutes.
3. Add rice.
4. Beat egg with tamari soy sauce and toasted sesame oil. Pour mixture into the pan and spread it around pan quickly to cook.
5. Lower heat and cool for 5 minutes more, stirring occasionally. Enjoy!

Black Bean & Corn Salad

Cilantro-Cumin Dressing

- 1/4 cup chopped, fresh cilantro
- 5 tablespoons olive oil
- 1/4 cup red wine vinegar
- 1 teaspoon ground cumin

Ingredients for bean salad to toss with dressing:

- 1 can (16 ounces) black beans, drained and rinsed
- 1 can (11 ounces) whole-kernel corn, drained
- 1 green pepper, diced
- 1 red bell pepper, diced
- 1 cup thinly sliced celery
- 1 cup thinly sliced green onions

Directions:

1. Combine the beans, corn, green pepper, bell pepper, celery, green onions and cilantro in a large mixing bowl.
2. Whisk the oil, vinegar and cumin in a separate smaller bowl. Pour the dressing over the vegetables and stir until thoroughly coated.
3. Let stand 15 minutes to blend the flavors, or refrigerate up to 2 hours before serving.

Oatmeal Pancakes

Ingredients:
- 1 ½ cup oatmeal
- ½ cup whole wheat
- 2 teaspoon baking powder
- 2 teaspoon cinnamon
- 1 tablespoon nut butter
- 1 banana, chopped
- 1 ¼ cup almond or rice milk

Directions:
1. Mix dry ingredients together in a medium size mixing bowl.
2. Add almond milk and mix.
3. Add nut butter and banana to mixture.
4. Lightly grease pan with olive or canola oil and turn on medium heat.
5. Pour batter into small round pancakes and heat until batter is fully cooked or when sides are golden brown. Enjoy!

Step 17

Discover the Void Behind Your Eating

The first thing people want to do when they gain weight is crash diet. Hoping to lose the most weight with the least amount of time and effort, many turn to promises of quick fixes. If quick fix diets worked, America would be the trimmest country in the world! Everyone would be walking around vibrantly and full of life. However, we are in an obesity crisis in the United States, and many struggle with weight, diabetes, high blood pressure, and other ailments excess weight causes.

As you think about how you eat currently, think back to any broken feelings or emotions of hurt, neglect, anger, or resentment.

Were you picked on as a kid, and cookies were your comfort? Think back. Then think about the present. Is something bothering you today and driving you to crave a certain food?

Food habits are often connected to past or present hurts. Ignoring or masking these issues will only cause more pain, heartache, addiction, and possible weight gain in the future. As hard as it hurts sometimes, we need to bring the motivation behind our food habits to the surface. As a recovering binge and emotional eater, I constantly have to keep myself in check. People might assume I have it all together, but the truth is, I re-read this book constantly because there are definitely days that I struggle!

A couple months ago, I returned home from a really awesome day—lots of wonderful things had happened, and my business seemed to be booming. I remember how great I felt and how happy I was. I got home early to cook a wonderful, nutritious meal and take some time for myself to relax.

At around 8 p.m. that night, however, I found myself headed for the fridge. I wasn't hungry, nor was I upset or bored. I stopped just as the refrigerator door was about to open and said, *"Wait, what do you really want? You had an awesome day? You had a wonderful filling meal? What could you possibly be hungry for?"* The truth is—I had no one to share my wonderful day with. I wasn't looking for comfort in calories, but instead, I just wanted someone to talk to—to hear me out, to share my excitement.

Happy as I was that day, there was a feeling of loneliness. I'm single, live alone, and am constantly listening to others throughout the day. So when I got home, good day and all, I wanted to share my day with another person. Recognizing that deep desire helped me shift my emotional junk food habit to the real life nourishment—calling a friend! This craving for companionship is universal, and it is often interpreted and nurtured in the wrong way.

~~~~~~~~~~ Keep Going ~~~~~~~~~~

So skip the fad diet and spend your energy discovering why you are eating in a certain way. Once you know why you eat, you can look for healthy ways to make new habits.

Ask yourself these questions:

- Do I go to the fridge when I'm not hungry?

- Do I eat when I'm bored?

- Do I get a sense of satisfaction from eating certain foods?

- Do I ever feel badly about eating foods I know I shouldn't be eating?

If you answer "yes" to any of these questions, this is a first step in raising your awareness. Now start to notice what role your food habit plays in your life over the next week. Why are you making certain food choices? What situation or circumstance is occurring when you see yourself heading to the fridge or drive-thru? What is the motivating force behind your choices? This force might be much deeper than you think.

Personal Story - A Step Along the Way
(I am not sharing this to brag or boast, but to make a point.)

I stepped on the scale recently to find myself five pounds lighter than normal. Then, when I went to the department store, I found myself fitting into smaller sized jeans than I'd ever fit into before.

I haven't changed my diet. In fact, I even splurged a few weeks prior and had pumpkin pie. Since dessert isn't my thing, this was huge for me. I have even been traveling a lot this past month, which also forces me to eat out. Again, something I rarely do. Despite all this, I lost weight.

So what's the secret? What's the quick fix? What diet pill was I taking?

The truth is—my nourishment this past month was not coming in the physical form of food. Other things have been *"feeding"* me this month: my career is right on point, my existing relationships are improving, new relationships are starting, and my spiritual side is affirming.

These non-food factors feed me. So at the end of my days, rather than heading to the kitchen for a late night snack, I feel full from the day's events or activities. People, places, connections, inspirations, and ideas all feed me. When I feel full and nourished, I don't need to seek out calories.

Take a minute and ask yourself, "What's feeding me?"
What can you do to truly feel whole and nourished
in all aspects of life, not simply in your belly?

Step 18
Drink More Water

Okay, so this is not exactly a new, breakthrough piece of advice. You've already been advised to increase the amount of water you drink before. Even so, you would be surprised at how many of us are actually dehydrated. Dehydration can cause massive problems with digestion, inflammation, headaches, hunger pains, and other health problems. In addition to keeping you hydrated, water flushes toxins from your system and helps you feel refreshed overall. Water is critical to feeling well.

Be more conscious of how much water you actually consume. Then try to increase that amount. You might begin by taking a water bottle to work and filling it up throughout the day. Invest in a reusable water bottle and make a commitment to use it.

Don't like the taste of water? Try adding lemon, lime, cucumber, or fruit slices to water for a naturally sweeter kick!

~~~~~ Keep Going ~~~~~

Challenge yourself: Drink one glass of water when you first wake up. Then continue throughout the day. It is easier to get into the groove of drinking water if you start your morning off drinking a full glass. How many glasses of water can you increase today? How about in five days? Start small and work your way up throughout the week!

Step 19
Slow Down

In today's fast-paced society, it is easy to feel rushed during every minute of the day. Most of us are constantly on the run and barely get a minute for ourselves. When it comes to food, we now have fast food, frozen dinners, and pre-made salad mix. We eat meals in our cars, on the couch, and on our 30-minute lunch breaks. Sit-down family dinners seem to be a thing of the past, and fast food makes it easier and more convenient to get a quick meal. Because of these elements in our culture, we often feel forced to eat our meals quickly so we can get to our next project.

Next time you eat a meal, slow things down. Take one bite, put your utensil down, and chew thoroughly. Really taste what you are eating. Enjoy every crunch, chew, and swallow. A lot of foods are sweeter than you'd expect when you take time to chew them fully. When you slow down the rate at which you eat, you will also feel full faster, so you'll be less tempted to over-eat.

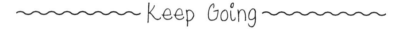

Keep Going

Plan out a day or two this week when you are going to *"slow it down."* Notice any change. Did you eat more, the same, or less? Did the food taste differently? How did you feel? Take notes. Remember—this is all for your benefit!

Feed Your Body - Quick Nourishing Tips:

- Treat your body like a test lab! After you eat, ask yourself, *"How do I feel?"*

- Remember, small changes = big results.

- Add color to your plate. See how many colors you can eat a day.

- Drink more water. Simple enough.

- Look for sweetness in non-food areas of your life.

6

Feeding Your Spirit

Love Yourself

"There are no extra pieces in the universe. Everyone is here because he or she has a place to fill, and every piece must fit itself into the big jigsaw puzzle."

~ Deepak Chopra

Step 20

Find Your Own God, Universe, or Buddha

Recently, at a family reunion, one of my cousins said, *"I found God through gardening."* However you find God, the Universe, or your inner peace—whether it's through gardening, biking, writing, or going to church—connect with something higher than yourself that calms you and makes you feel whole. Build a relationship with your higher power, and nurture that relationship on a regular basis. This relationship will help you stay calm, cool, and collected during stressful times.

You're Almost There

Here are three easy ways to connect with a higher power or engage in a spiritual practice:

1. **Get quiet.** Take time for silence and stillness each day. Let your mind rest and get into a meditative state. Try to void out all the day-to-day clutter in your head, even if for a few minutes out of the day. This practice will help ease your mind and sooth your inner world.

2. **Surround yourself with like-minded people.** Remember, *"Like attracts like."* If you want to feel positive and upbeat, surround yourself with positive, upbeat people. Relationships with optimistic people help lift your spirit and can shift your energy dramatically.

3. **Explore!** Take time to explore different churches, retreats, meditations, readings, yoga practices, art, music, and more. See what starts feeling right for you and explore it more deeply.

Step 21
Be Present

Did you ever drive to a destination and, upon arriving, couldn't remember exactly how you got there? Did you ever listen to someone else talking only to realize later that you had no idea what that person was talking about? We are so focused on our fast-paced lives that we often forget to pay attention to the world around us. We rush by signs, nature, houses, and people without blinking an eye.

On a day-to-day basis, we let many of life's natural beauties fly by us. We forget how fresh air smells or how beautiful the tree in our own backyard is. We forget to embrace the gifts that surround us. Our fast-paced lifestyles obscure our experiences of fresh fallen leaves, the song of a blue bird, or the breeze in our hair. These wonders go unnoticed. As a consequence, our deepest spirits go unnourished.

Start by simply being present in your own life. Find peace and joy in nature and your surroundings. Smile at someone walking down the hall or the sidewalk. Simply put, just be.

Appreciate the current moment for what it is, right now. Make stopping to appreciate a moment a discipline in your life.

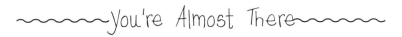

Challenge yourself with this exercise:

Take a mindful walk.

- Walk slowly.

- Stop.

- Look at the intricate details in your surroundings.

- See the veins on leaves, the insects crawling on trees, and the different colors in front of you.

- Now hear the birds chirping, the wind blowing in the background, or the crinkle of leaves beneath animal feet.

- Stop once again. Would you have noticed these things if you had not made the effort to be present?

Did you ever drive to a destination and, upon arriving, you couldn't remember the exactly how you got there? Simply start being present in your own life. Find peace and joy in nature and your surroundings. Smile at someone walking down the hall or the sidewalk. Simply, just be.

Step 22
Act Like a Kid Again

Laugh, giggle, chuckle, snicker, hoot, or holler. Whatever you call it—do it. Relax, have fun, and remember to laugh. Laughing reduces stress tremendously and helps get you in a better frame of mind.

Babies and children constantly laugh. As we get older, however, we are told to be more serious, to stop with the nonsense. This admonition, repeated over time, leads us to get so serious that we forget to open ourselves to joy and laughter.

The feeling of awe and excitement children get during traditional holidays is unlike any other. I still remember the feeling I had as a child—the anticipation, the curiosity, and the thrill of waking up on Christmas morning to find presents under the tree and half-eaten cookies Santa left behind. The mystery, wonder, and fascination seemed to overtake my imagination.

The littlest things about the holidays gave us great joy as children. We felt no judgment from the outside world to squash our joy. We simply lived in the present moment, feeling excited about life, and enjoying our very being.

As we got older, however, Christmas seemed to change. Suddenly, the lights on the Christmas tree meant less, we stopped putting out cookies for Santa, and the anticipation dwindled. Christmas started to lose its magic. Why does our joy around Christmas and other holidays diminish as adults? Is it because we know the *"truth"* about Santa, or is it because Christmas starts to feel like a stressful chore? Either way, our once magical Christmas slowly loses the spark.

Unfortunately, we don't just lose the magic during Christmas or significant holidays, we also lose the magic in other instances in our lives as well. We lose the magic or spark in our relationships, our careers, and ourselves.

~~~~~~~~~~~You're Almost There~~~~~~

Take some time this week to find the magic and awe you once had as a child. Start looking at things through the eyes of a child. Feed your spirit by putting on your favorite funny movie, looking up a funny video that may be new to you, or enjoying the company of funny people!

Let go of your *"serious"* mode for just a bit. Forget the outside stresses, and act like a kid again. Feel the excitement and joy in everyday living. After all, who said we need to act our age?

Suggestions to Re-capture your Childhood Magic

- Celebrate a friend, a significant other, or a family member. Think back to the time you first met. Think about how you felt around this person during the best of times. Relive those feelings, even if only for a few moments.

- Make smiley face pancakes for breakfast.

- Watch a Disney classic—take yourself back to your favorite childhood movie. Remember how you used to feel watching it? Capture these feelings again.

- Simply smile and laugh. Don't take life too seriously.

Step 23
Breathe

Did you ever have one of those crazy, off-the-wall days where you get home and ask yourself, *"Wait, what just happened? Where did the day go?"* Once again, our fast-paced society is the culprit. We *"run, run, run"* all day, every day—so much that we tense up, take shallow breaths, and get winded walking up a flight of stairs.

During the next week or so, take time to breathe. Enough said. Just take a second to breathe.

The simple practice of noticing your breath can help you relax and slow down. Once this becomes a habit, you might want to take this activity to the next step and practice deep breathing.

～～～You're Almost There～～～

To practice deep breathing:

- Lie flat on your back with your hands on your stomach.

- Breathe in deeply until you feel your stomach expand.

- Hold for ten seconds.

- Breathe out and let your stomach shrink in.

- Repeat five times.

Notice your breath, and notice how your muscles tense less when you practice breathing deeply. Practice this exercise every day for the next week, especially if you find yourself in stressful situations. What happens to your feelings of stress or anxiety? Do they subside more when you practice breathing deeply? Keep practicing—the results only get better!

Everyone encounters this thing called anxiety at some time or another. However, the second we let words like anxiety and depression define who we are, is the day we put a block against our authentic self. Rather than having this term define you, instead, re-define yourself--the real authentic you. Shed the label and be you!

Step 24

Recognize Your Unique Beauty

"I'm too fat. My *nose is too big. My lips are uneven. My ears look like elephant ears."* The list goes on and on and on. . .

Learn to fall in love with you. Treat yourself with the same dignity, respect, and love with which you treat others you care about. Learn to love your features. If you have curvy hips, embrace them. If you have skinny legs, love them.

During my years of intense anxiety, I never left the house without makeup. I thought I was ugly and needed to *"doll up"* every day. My best friend was stick-figure skinny, so on top of the need for makeup, I was self-conscious about my weight. I had a persistently negative view of my body.

However, once my health changed, I began to realize my unique beauty, and guess what? So did everyone else. When I felt better about myself, I became more confident in my own skin and others took notice. I didn't necessarily lose a ton of weight or stop wearing makeup. I did, however, begin to portray a confidence that indicated, *"Yes, I love who I am and yes, I treat myself with respect."*

Rather than spending time stressing and complaining about features you perceive to be negative, learn to love and embrace your uniqueness. I learned to love my stick-thin legs, my thick arms, my wide nose, and my big feet. These features are what make me . . . well, me!

~~~~~You're Almost There~~~~~

What qualities make you amazing, inside and out? Embrace those qualities by recording them below. When you aren't feeling so good about yourself, look back on your list and remember all your beautiful qualities.

I am amazing because:_____

_____

_____

_____

Step 25

Take the Grateful Challenge

There is no better feeling than appreciating and being grateful for what is already yours.

How many times have you heard someone say, *"My car broke down, I don't have any money, my boyfriend just broke up with me, and to top it off, now I'm sick."* We tend to get bogged down by negativity and forget to stop and appreciate the many things in our lives we can be happy for. Even in trying circumstances, we need to be grateful and ask ourselves what lessons we are being taught. Sometimes we might not see the lesson right away, but there is always a reason for the circumstances that enter our lives.

Start each new day by being grateful for waking up, breathing, and being here now. Write down the things you are truly grateful for each day. As you make this a daily practice, you might be amazed at how many more things you are grateful for!

~~~~You're Almost There~~~~

Take the one-week gratitude challenge: In a journal record five things you are grateful for every morning or every evening. As the week progresses, you might notice that the practice gets easier and more joyful. If you have a hard time thinking of five things, then start with two or three. Don't worry about repeating yourself either.

We can be grateful for the same things everyday. At the end of the week you may ask yourself, *"Why stop at just five things?"* Start now!

Today, I am grateful for:

1. _____

2. _____

3. _____

4. _____

5. _____

Step 26

Confront Your Negative Seeds and Weeds

Children feel invincible, carefree, and are apt to say whatever is on their minds. They truly love themselves. As children start to grow and develop motor skills, they start to understand the world around them. They start to notice when other people approve and disapprove of them. With this, children also start to experience the negative emotions that come with self-consciousness.

Each of us, as growing children, experienced someone sneaking up on us and planting a negative seed, causing weeds of self-doubt to grow around us. We shrunk, at least a little, and the weeds took root. Over time, we forgot we have the power to pull out the weeds to see the beautiful flower or garden—the garden that happens to be us.

One negative seed, especially if that seed is nurtured over time, can be enough to devastate us. My clients often share instances they remember as children or teens that have been implanted in them. These individuals have lived their entire lives accepting their negative seed, allowing weeds to sprout until, eventually, even the sun becomes shaded by the enormous weeds.

Negative seeds are often hurtful words or experiences. Here are examples people have shared with me.

- Being called *"fatso"* by your father at age seven

- Being called a *"slut"* at age thirteen

- Being called *"ugly"* in sixth grade

- Or yes, even your parents missing your first play in fourth grade

Criticisms, being abandoned or treated as second best, and other negative experiences, remain visually and emotionally present in people's lives for years on end. Even if the person doesn't dwell on the pain often, the related feelings stay stored in the subconscious. Many people don't realize their negative seeds of self-doubt and even self-loathing were planted in them from the outside, often at a tender age. Without awareness, some people spend their whole lives living out a lie someone has told them about themselves. They become the mature version of the negative seed. If we let negative seeds manifest who we are, we limit our chances to live happy and abundant lives.

Recognizing that others have planted negative seeds in you is the first step towards transformation. Acknowledge and identify each seed, but realize that a negative seed has no power to determine who you are. You are yourself, and only you have the right to decide who you are, inside and out. Remember these words from Eleanor Roosevelt, *"No one has the power to make you feel inferior without your permission."*

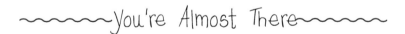

You're Almost There

Start today and just say, *"No!"* to negative voices and seeds, past or present. Do not let anyone else have the power to define you, your attitude, or your inner being.

Ask yourself, *"Who am I really?"* Write your answer out. Take a minute to write out all the positive qualities you can identify about yourself. *(Remember, only you have the right to decide who you are!)*

I am: _____

_____

_____

_____

_____

_____

_____

_____

Step 27
Plant Happy Seeds

Have you ever noticed how we vividly remember criticism while quickly forgetting sincere compliments? Everyone shares this tendency.

We feed our own spirits and make the world a better place when we radiate and plant happy seeds in others. Compliment your neighbor. Sow a kind word. Bring a snack to share at work. Buy someone's dinner. A little deed of kindness and affirmation can create a domino effect in someone's life, bringing happiness. When you plant happy seeds with others, you will end up receiving happy seeds right back. This is a law of the universe. Plant happy seeds in others: you might just be surprised at how full your own garden grows!

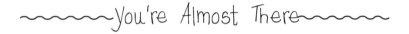

You're Almost There

Here are some suggestions to get you started, but remember to use your creativity and make this practice authentic to you! Use the space at the end to add your own ideas.

- Buy a stranger coffee when you find yourself in a line.

- Put a quarter in a meter that is about to expire.

- Smile at a stranger.

- Tip a server generously.

- Donate to your favorite charity.

- Compliment someone in the checkout line.

- Volunteer at a local shelter.

- Hold the door for someone.

- Offer advice to a friend.

- Invite someone to cut in front of you at the grocery store.

- Donate blood.

- _____.

- _____.

- _____.

- _____.

- _____.

- _____.

Feed Your Spirit - Quick Inspiring Tips:

- Stop and be present to the world around you.

- Act like a kid! Do something that makes you feel alive and young again.

- Breathe, simply breathe.

- Tell yourself why you are amazing.

- Ask yourself daily, *"What am I grateful for?"*

- Make someone's day and the gesture will make your day too.

7

The Airport Stranger Revisited

Trust Your Journey and Embrace the Small Steps

It's been a long time since an encounter with a stranger in an airport shifted my perspective on healthy living and filled me with new compassion and understanding. I've never forgotten the lesson I learned that day: the relationship each of us has with food is much more than calorie deep. Our foods and our moods do an intricate dance throughout our lives. Typically, junk foods are related to junk moods in one way or another in a vicious cycle. Here's the good news: you can interrupt the cycle and choose a healthy lifestyle.

Losing weight, eating in healthy ways, and finding balance are not things you can achieve with quick fixes. Discovering yourself and unraveling your habits around food involves a process, not a single "aha" moment or epiphany. Reaching a true sense of well-being in mind, body, and spirit takes time, patience, and a whole lot of soul-searching. This is a process of growing, learning from past circumstances, and overcoming trying times to shape yourself into the person you want to be.

Even when the anxiety I experienced as a child diminished and I began to feel better, I still didn't fully understand what led me to choose the foods I did. I slipped into old habits sometimes, and then I started eating in healthy ways again—but I didn't address my underlying issues. In fact, I didn't even know I had underlying issues that were related to my habits around food.

Over the years, as I became more aware of myself, including my mind, my body, and my spirit, I was able to dig a little deeper to discover the true issues behind my eating habits. And that's when true breakthroughs began to occur.

My goal in writing this book has been to raise your consciousness when it comes to your food habits. To repeat myself, food is usually much more than calorie deep; our relationship with food is deeply emotional. To put it simply, when we crave junky foods, it's often because we feel junky about ourselves in some way. The answer, of course, isn't to eat junky food; the answer lies in getting to the root of our junky feelings.

If you are struggling with weight and unhealthy food choices, chances are the foods you choose are filling a void for you. A big step toward change is to identify that void and to process your feelings about it. Another big step is to develop the habit of treating your body like a lab. Pay attention to the foods you eat and how your body feels after eating those foods. Observe the personal dance you have with foods and moods.

While the good news is that you can interrupt a negative cycle among foods and moods, the bad news is that you can't rush things. You must learn to take smalls steps and build upon small successes. Never beat yourself up because you haven't conquered your food problems in a jiffy.

At the same time, don't give up. This book is meant to "feed" you for a long time. Consume it slowly, and chew on each individual step for as long as needed. Choose a step to implement during a week, two weeks, or even a month. As the initial changes you make become incorporated into your routine, try adding another small change from another tip. Remember, you are embarking on a process and a journey to a lifetime of health, not a crash diet that will begin and end in a month.

Trust your journey, and embrace the wisdom of small steps. You CAN break the cycle of junk foods and junk moods!

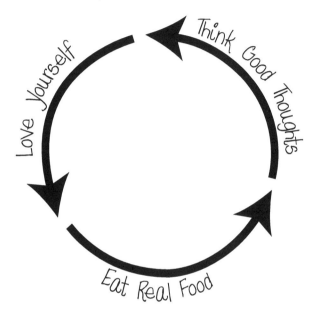

~~~~~~~~Repeat As Needed~~~~~~~~

Love Yourself

Think Good Thoughts

Eat Real Food

Remember you are embarking on a lifetime journey. Events and situations happen that can cause us to be out of balance in one or all three areas of the mind, body, and spirit. Use this book as often as you need. Start in the section that needs the most healing and continue to repeat as necessary!

About The Author

Lindsey Smith

Lindsey Smith began her cycle of binge eating at age 4. Her foods of choice were Swedish Goldfish, Watermelon Sour Patch Gummies, and blue Flying Saucers. With a background like that, you can count on Lindsey to demonstrate compassion and humor as well as powerful insights into your relationship with food.

After overcoming childhood anxiety and weight gain through discovering the connection between foods and moods, Lindsey immersed herself in studying the emotional connections people have with food. She learned that when people look to food for nutrients like acceptance, comfort, celebration, and love, a disastrous cycle of junk foods and junk moods begins. This insight, combined with Lindsey's expertise as a certified Health Coach, means Lindsey is ideally qualified to help clients gain freedom over destructive food habits.

Founder of *"The Real You,"* Lindsey serves clients as a keynote speaker, a one-on-one coach, and author of the book Junk Foods and Junk Moods. (launch date is set for January 2012) She helps clients lose weight, increase energy, and gain a healthy lifestyle by uncovering their personal connection with the foods they eat and their moods.

Lindsey's approach is not a quick-fix, quick-fail diet, but rather a journey toward understanding yourself and the food choices you make. Her solutions are not designed to make clients sacrifice or deprive themselves for health, but to make small changes that build to big results.

Whether you work with Lindsey one-on-one, engage her to deliver a presentation, or read Junk Foods and Junk Moods, you can be sure you will laugh, cry, and find inspiring solutions to your own problems with food and mood relationships!

Invite Lindsey to Speak to
Your Group or Organization

Lindsey is a dynamic and powerful speaker on the topics of: nutrition, healthy lifestyle, dreaming big, attitude, and overcoming obstacles.

Lindsey's enthusiasm, passion for life, and even the ability to stand before a crowd, wasn't always the case. After a series of internal struggles and traumas, Lindsey realized at a young age that she had a choice—a choice to choose a better way of living.

Lindsey takes her audiences on a journey—from the struggle and despair to hope and healing. She gives them not only the motivation, but she also gives them the tools to achieve a life of health and happiness.

Her humor, personal stories, and motivation has been a crowd pleaser to many audiences including:

- The Pennsylvania Nutrition Education Network
- The Pennsylvania Mental Health Consumer Association
- Community Action Southwest
- Alle-Kiski Health Foundation
- Women's Business Network Annual Retreat
- Westchester Association for the Education of Young Children
- …and many more

Rave Reviews!

"In Junk Foods and Junk Moods, Lindsey Smith takes readers on an introspective journey behind the scenes of one's lifestyle choices, uncovering the important connection between nutrition, thought patterns and emotional wellness. With this awareness, one becomes powerfully equipped to make new and better choices that support greater health and happiness. Junk Foods and Junk Moods is a must-read for anyone looking to thrive physically, mentally and emotionally in today's world."

~Lorraine Miller
Author of From Gratitude to Bliss:
A Journey in Health and Happiness, nourishbynature.com

"My experience with The Real You and Lindsey Smith was fantastic. In 6 weeks, I not only learned a better way to feed my body, gaining energy and stamina, I also lost at least one pant and 2 dress sizes. I feel that these classes put myself and my family on the right path to start 2012 healthier, happier and in more control of the choices that we make when it comes to what feeds us – including the "primary foods" of our relationships, careers, and physical activity. I would recommend the 6 Week Weight Loss Program to anyone who is ready to take control of these things and come out more content – and skinnier! – on the other side!"

~Symone Ciencin, 6-Week Weight Loss Program

"That was eye-opening for me. To see that you could confidently stand there and say that you had a problem and you are ok now gave me a sense of hope that I haven't felt in awhile. I thought that I was going to the meeting to pick up a few tid bits about nutrition and it ended up being so much more. Thank you. Your passion for what you do is so apparent and motivating!"

~Nicole, Women's Health Workshop

"The work that Lindsey does puts her on the forefront of this field and allows her to help people in a very unique way. The services she provides tap into aspects of individuals that most others do not consider important to health. This opens their eyes to the "cure" they've been searching for, and improves people's entire beings to provide them with a happier life. Lindsey has been a tremendous friend to me and is helping me become a person that I can truly be happy about. I can't imagine not having her, or her services, available to me."

~Kristen, Dental Student

For More Products & Services Visit:

www.FoodMoodGirl.com

www.TheRealYouNutrition.com

Connect With Lindsey!

info@foodmoodgirl.com

www.FoodMoodGirl.com

www.Facebook.com/FoodMoodGirl

www.Facebook.com/TheRealYouNutrition

www.Twitter.com/LindseySmithHHC

www.YouTube.com/TheRealYouNutrition

Made in the USA
Charleston, SC
15 April 2014